Communication in health care

*Understanding and implementing
effective human relationships*

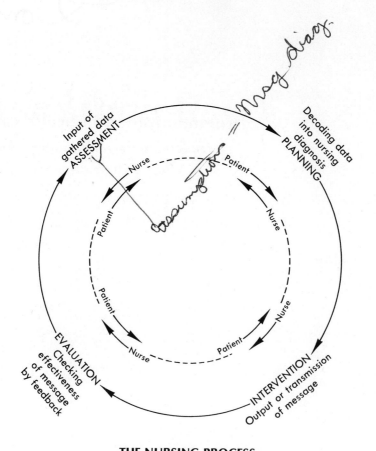

THE NURSING PROCESS
Dynamic link in the chain of communication

Communication
in health care

*Understanding and implementing
effective human relationships*

Mattie Collins, R.N., B.S., M.A.

Associate Professor, Department of Nursing,
Borough of Manhattan Community College,
New York, New York

The C. V. Mosby Company

Saint Louis   1977

The C. V. Mosby Company
11830 Westline Industrial Drive, St. Louis, Missouri 63141

Library of Congress Cataloging in Publication Data

Collins, Mattie, 1929-
    Communication in health care.

    Bibliography: p.
    Includes index.
    1. Nurse and patient.   2. Communication in nursing.
3. Interpersonal communication.   4. Nursing ethics.
I. Title.   [DNLM: 1. Communication.   2. Nurse-
patient relations.   3. Delivery of health care.   WY87
C712c]
RT86.C63   610.73′01′9   76-30551
ISBN 0-8016-1021-4

TS/M/M   9   8   7   6   5   4   3   2   1

To
Mother
Rudy
Terry
Keely
Kim
and the rest of the family,
who verbally and nonverbally
communicated love

Preface

The purpose of this book is to assist in the transfer of theoretical concepts concerning human relationships to the reality of people care. It is written for those who are learning to be people helpers and those who wish to learn more about the art of helping people. The essence of any helping process is communication; a significant correlation appears to exist between problems in human relationships and problems in communication. This book is a response to the many requests by students for resource material to help them deal with psychodynamic situations, sociopsychologic problems, and communication questions (judgmental test items) in clinical practice and theoretical problem solving.

The various labels that students applied to their concerns indicated that they were using familiar terms to render comprehensible some rather elusive body of knowledge concerning basic interpersonal relationships. Their difficulty prompted referrals to the many current texts on the subject in nursing and other related disciplines. However, such referrals did not satisfy what seemed to be an insatiable thirst for knowledge. Their perception of the problem was that too many texts stressed the "why to" and the "what to" often at the expense of the "how to," when such processes must be synergistic if a relationship is to have meaning.

I view theoretical knowledge as the "why" and technical competence as the "what" of the helping process; but this is not enough. For example, a nurse alone with a patient needing artificial respiration may well know *what* should be done and the scientific *whys* for doing so. However, if she has neglected *how* to proceed, all the concepts, principles, and theories that she has mastered concerning the effects of sustained oxygen deprivation on living organisms will be of no benefit to the patient. Although knowledge and skill are vital blocks in building human relationships, something must fix or hold these elements together. They resist transformation into supportive care. Communication is the essential cement in human relationships, binding the blocks together. It is the "how to" of interpersonal relationships: how to reach out to and be reached by one another. This book is one means of demonstrating to the student a congruence between the what, why, and how of a therapeutic relationship.

Readers are not expected to master the material in this book as if they were assimilating concrete facts from a discipline such as anatomy or physiology. It is a proved fact that man has one brain with three primary divisions: forebrain, midbrain, and hindbrain. Each individual, however, differs in emotions, attitudes, imagination, thoughts, feelings, and reasoning patterns—those parts which form the "relatedness" of interactions with others. The infinite variety and complexity of human responses limit the helper's reliance on concise, definitive theoretical concepts and infallible, verifiable techniques. Man is a capricious animal and does not readily surrender his sovereignty of self to specific scientific formulations.

The book has two major divisions. The first is a discussion of conceptual frameworks thought to have relevance to helping relationships. It is an attempt to clarify theoretical formulations. The elaboration of theoretical concepts has a dual purpose: to present guidelines to maximize the potential of actual helping relationships and to assist in transfer of knowledge to the hypothetical situations that comprise the second part of the book, which is even more ambitious. It is an attempt to make theoretical formulations practical. The hypothetical situations derive from living and learning. Analysis of the various responses represents a personal synthesis of many schools of thought. Explanatory points of view serve only as guidelines: in a particular situation the tentative application of a particular principle might be the most helpful. Guidelines chart uncertain courses; they should not be considered error-free maps. Readers must decide for themselves the best course to pursue in helping others.

This book will also help beginning practitioners to fulfill expanded roles in caring for persons in a variety of settings. How? Instructors may find the book useful as a supplementary text in whatever area interpersonal relationships are taught. It could also be used to enhance teaching methodologies as a source for role-playing situations and patient-study discussions.

Students who were exposed to samples of the material in the second part of the book often heatedly differed with me. More importantly the material was found to provide relevant stimuli for further discussion of situations that occurred in their own clinical experiences and thus to reinforce the applicability of classroom learning to practice. If you, the readers, similarly respond, the purpose of this book will have been more than fulfilled.

For the sake of expedience rather than any chauvinistic intent, the term *nurse* usually refers to the feminine gender and *patient* to the male. Females, as well as males, are included in the terms *man* and *mankind.*

Although the word *client* is now often used for *patient,* I have kept the time-honored term *patient* both because it may be more familiar to readers and because it implies a closer relationship.

Don't be discouraged if the cement of human relationships flakes and crumbles. Keep trying. Make some new mortar. With practice you will build an edifice uniquely your own.

Mattie Collins

Contents

Communication in health care

*Understanding and implementing
effective human relationships*

PART ONE

Concepts
related to communication

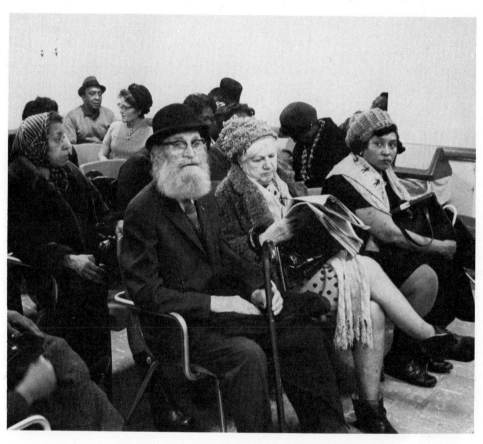

Americans value sociability. Synonymous with sociability is communication—the matrix of contemporary society. Communication forges the link between man and man—between man and groups. Missing links may be noticeable when cultural differences complicate the communication network. Missing links may lead to anomie; human beings become detached from and not available to or deeply aware of others. (Photograph by Bruce Anspach, Editorial Photocolor Archives.)

CHAPTER 1

The communication process

OVERVIEW

Despite such elaborate terminology as *team nursing, primary nursing, nursing diagnosis, nursing hypothesis,* and *nursing intervention,* more than ten years of experience as a visiting nurse in New York have shown me that few specific care functions ordinarily assigned to the nurse cannot be carried out by others. Instead nursing is defined with its patient-interaction process as a critical point.

Families have adapted many nursing activities to the home environment, retaining autonomy of attitudes, beliefs, customs, and values. Nurses have taught self-care to patients or family members within a variety of cultural and social patterns. Diabetic children with language barriers have been taught to give their own injections and to test their urine. Lay persons have learned to supervise medication and dietary regimens; to suction tracheotomies and to remove, cleanse, and reinsert the inner cannula; to irrigate any cavity at the direction of a physician; to assess vital signs with mastery of the mystique of the sphygmomanometer; to use respirators; to apply hot and cold compresses; and to use sterile techniques in changing dressings on any anatomic structure within their reach. Many homes were visited for what was broadly categorized as *health supervision* with opportunities for individuals to identify their problems and become actively involved in the nursing assessment, planning, implementation, and evaluation of care. Members of the community were found capably carrying out "nursing" tasks: grandparents were found supervising the new teenage mother; members of halfway houses were found supervising drug addicts; and landlords of single-room–occupancy buildings were found supervising the health, hospitalization, and sometimes burial of social isolates. One may conclude that many persons without formal credentials can and do care for, comfort, and meet the needs of individuals in their communities.

Although aiding others is not the special prerogative of any group, nursing is an *especially* helpful activity. The essence of this special activity is the nature of the interpersonal relationship, since nursing is based on helping, and development of interpersonal relationships is basic to nursing. The nurse is the one member of the health team who is readily accessible in many settings to give sustained personal service to an individual undergoing a major or minor life change. The nurse is available for the short moments and the long days. Basic to this interpersonal relationship is the quality of communication between nurses, patients, families, and other members of the health team. Communication is essential to assistance:

> . . . assisting the individual, sick or well, in the performance of those activities contributing to health or its recovery (or to a peaceful death) that he would perform unaided if he had the necessary strength, will or knowledge. And to do so in such a way as to help him gain independence as soon as possible.[1]

Communication is not just the kind that takes place over an intercom system between nurses' stations and the patients' units. Communication in nursing is much more: the purposeful and humane implementation of knowledge in face-to-face relationships with mutual involvement of participants in the problem-solving process.

TRENDS IN NURSING THAT AFFECT COMMUNICATION

In the quest for professional status, in nursing the "doing" components have been undervalued, and the managerial aspects of practice have been stressed.[2] To some extent this view reflects the societal evaluation of manual work, which unless highly specialized or dramatic is less esteemed than managerial work. Nurses who have the broadest educational exposure to the behavioral sciences have become overseers instead of givers of service. In contrast, the ministering roles tend to be filled by those who are the least prepared from the standpoint of formal education. Not surprisingly, such roles hold low status in terms of the societal rewards of earnings, prestige, and privileges. "In addition to our tendency to value managerial skills very highly, we have a tendency to use words rather imprecisely and, at times with a little pomposity."[2] The nonprofessional givers of direct patient care are said to be extensions of the nurse—her "arms" and "ears." To make this so magically, we have titled them *nursing assistants.*

The nonprofessionals are not to be disparaged: they function well on their levels of competence; but the well-fed and refreshed patient in a tidy unit often becomes "difficult"—lonely, fearful, and anxious. Needs are communicated through intermediaries, and much can be lost in the transmission and translation of the message. Covert concerns may be interpreted as overt complaints. Indirect nursing care makes it difficult to see the individual as more than pieces of reported behaviors.

Kramer describes the phenomenon of "reality shock" in the new graduate nurse as a result of the "startling discovery and reaction to the discovery that school-bred values conflict with work-world values."[3] A sharp discontinuity is perceived between the professional role concept of caring for and meeting the needs of the patient as a whole and the bureaucratic concept of segmented and technical patient care. The disenchantment between what the nurse learned was good and valued and what she now finds is the way things are done can "lead to less professionalism with continued employment."[4]

In some occupational settings the production of services tends to be organized on the same basis as the production of goods, and work output is "judged in terms of units completed."[5] Definite ideas exist concerning the characteristics of good nurses. The characteristics are limited mostly to what is directly observable and documented. Evaluation of the outcome of nursing care is partly in terms of adherence to defined procedural rules and regulations. Prudence and discretion, not valor, are the measure and the rule of those who seek to nurse. Indeed, such conforming behavior must show up with regularity in nurses' evaluations if they are to be promoted or to retain their jobs. The imperatives and priorities set in institutions can be strong determinants of the priorities set by nurses.

"Good nurses" are first of all economizers, especially with regard to time. They follow set routines, so that the most work can be done as efficiently as possible in the least amount of time. Observable tasks, such as treatments, medications, bathing, toileting, temperature taking, and bed making, are expected to be validated on patients' charts as having been completed on schedule. Time slots are provided for almost all such nursing activities. Paychecks are not given for "just sitting" or "just talking" with patients. Whatever interpersonal relationship develops in such circumscribed patient-care situations may be more incidental or accidental than planned.

In summary, these are issues that should be considered by those in the profession in planning for the future if not remedying the present. Certainly reality is painful. Certainly one's powers are limited. Certain problems may be insoluble. Despite this, a world of hope is found in *trying,* and perhaps that is all or almost all that any professional can do.

What cannot be changed outright can often be modified. Nurse administrators may work under conditions that make them less available to patients than they might desire, but the structure of the work situation should force nurses neither to lower nor to lose their ideals. Hence nurses have a dual responsibility to patients: to try to find out which patients need help and to match this need with the member of the health team most qualified to give such help. Those entrusted to give care should also be carefully supervised.

Similarly the profession needs more humanistic nurses. Initiative and thoughtful planning can do a great deal to make effective verbal and nonverbal communication a part of all nursing activities. Touching is an integral part of nursing intervention. The most basic nursing skills require touch. It is not only a means of establishing communication but also a vital way of communicating emotions and ideas. The comforting effects of touch are receiving increasing emphasis as important contributions to human well-being.[6] Much satisfaction can be gained in knowing that the judicious use of this form of communication facilitated the recovery process. Touching heals. Krieger[7] found in her research that as a result of the therapeutic laying on of hands, patients not only experienced a sense of relaxation and well-being but laboratory reports also demonstrated an increase in hemoglobin values. Highly motivated, healthy persons seem to have a natural potential to help or heal through therapeutic touch. Touching is an important nursing function that does not have to be reclaimed!

Just so, the nurse can use one activity that is familiar to patients as an adjunct to a somewhat unfamiliar one. For example, basic nursing skills combined with listening make nursing care comprehensive. Patients do not usually expect the nurse to truly listen. Barriers that make them hesitant to initiate or engage freely in communication are perceived. Believing that nurses are always busy and overworked, patients seem extremely reluctant to bother them with requests for information or services or with complaints.[8] In effective communication the nurse is "receiver oriented," as well as "message oriented." Patient feedback is a critical dimension in humanistic care.

COMMUNICATION: A FELT DIFFICULTY

The paradox that social trends toward specialization and generalization exist concurrently makes life interesting, challenging, and confusing and the implications for nursing profound. Consider specialization first.

The fallout from the age of specialization in the health professions is depersonalization. Man has been divided into physiologic and anatomic compartments, segments, quadrants, and sectors with licensed overseers for each part of his human form. The fact that his condition even warrants inspection by a specialist is disquieting to the individual from the start. He has learned or soon will learn that he should talk to the specialist concerning only that portion of his being which is the specialist's forte. For the patient to discuss the bunion on his toe with the cardiologist would be inappropriate, and the ophthalmologist would certainly view with a jaundiced eye any discussion of the patient's bowel functions.

However, man is more than systems and symptoms. One is unlikely to hear him say, "I am a heart condition." When he speaks of his illness, he is more likely to say, "I *have* a heart condition." He communicates to us that he is more than a disease entity and that he may need more than the treatment of his physical symptoms to get well. One of the most basic characteristics of man is his tendency to respond as a *whole:* a total, organized system, in which changes in any part may produce alterations in any other part. Human beings pursue wholeness and must be given opportunities to communicate their need for nursing intervention that preserves their sense of structural, spiritual, and personal intactness.

In microcosm, man is the social model of communication circuits, with intricate channels for receiving and responding to stimuli. That social stimulation is necessary for a healthy mind, as well as body, was documented by Spitz.[9] Children separated from their parents and reared in a foundling home demonstrated a "starvation syndrome," despite physical nourishment that was adequate in quality and quantity. The conclusion is inescapable: regardless of the adequacy of physical care, messages devoid of love and compassion can cause death or mental retardation in early life. Although the young are especially vulnerable, communications devoid of humaneness may cause states of disequilibrium in any part of the life cycle.

Why do former patients who have "recovered" often band together in such groups as mastectomy, colostomy, nephrostomy, and ileostomy clubs? Perhaps such self-help groups provide the kind of acceptance and sincerity needed for the communication of feelings and concerns associated with the specific disability and its consequences. This is not to say that the relationships such individuals had with nurses were less than satisfactory but rather to illustrate the pervasive need for communication and to focus attention on the many patients who are unable to meet their belonging and esteem needs within the supportive context of such groups. Unless nurses can establish relationships that better help patients to maintain unity, yet another specialist may be added to the health team. Is such a specialist the new employee in some institutions, the patient's advocate? Working on the patient's behalf, the advocate helps to solve problems encountered in health care situations when the patient feels that his own efforts are futile.

Together with specialization is the generalization to "massness." Things are being done in very large ways: mass media, mass transportation, mass defections, mass production, and mass meetings. The fallout is anomie.

Man begins to communicate at birth. Whether or not he cries, he transmits a message and receives attention. Man communicates at death. He transmits a message that either his heart or his brain has ceased functioning. He receives attention, but within this health-illness continuum, man is "conceived not as an individual" but as one of a multitude of persons in society—a mass man.[10] He is bombarded with signs and symbols that are mass produced and mass transmitted for the mass taste by the mass media. Having learned to tune in via television and Telestar to the opinions, values, and ideas of others in distant cities and countries, he has learned to "tune out" the opinions, values, and ideas of his neighbors. The extent of engineered messages pressing against one's senses is alarming. Toffler noted that in America the average adult is "assaulted by a minimum of 560 advertising messages each day" but only "notices 76."[11] This means that 484 messages are blocked out! The consequence is that too much irrelevant stimuli makes it easy to block out what is relevant. Simply too many waves of information are coming faster and faster, pounding like violent breakers for entry into one's nervous system.

The vicarious involvement with distant others has created social distance within society's basic unit: the family. Whole generations appear to have fallen into "gaps," and the credo of "togetherness," a valiant attempt to fill the void, is said to need the constant affirmation of family members' playing and praying in unison. Too many distractions make it difficult for man to concentrate on anyone for any length of time and to pay attention to what anyone is saying or not saying. Cues have become so ambiguous that one finds difficulty in telling whether a raised fist is a sign of wrath, victory, or brotherhood. He tends to mind his own business; he has made a virtue of uninvolvement. Specialization and generalization have made meaningful interactions uncommon. Since they are not the antithesis of each other, there are no inherent checks and balances for the progressive betterment of human relationships. Both social trends show scant regard for the value of uniqueness.

A literary resurgence of protest has appeared. Much has been written to help nurses to assist man to adjust not only to the changes within himself but to the rapid changes from without. The references in this chapter reflect the sheer diversity in the literature and the dimensions of the problem. However, a unifying theme can be found. We must begin to rethink our professional approach to helping: how to use our resources better for overcoming communication barriers to understanding and being understood.

COMMUNICATION: ART AND SCIENCE

Effective communication is not a natural consequence of the helping commitment. It is a worthwhile ideal, but the combination of art and science could help make the goal of effective communication more real. Although science has expanded the boundaries of human knowledge, human experience may resist codification in purely scientific formulations. Thus meaningful communication is a creative process, infusing knowledge and skill with feelings.

Art animates and accentuates human existence, providing the feeling tone for interpersonal relationships. Art stems from a basic emotional concern for and sensitivity to others. Sensitive, concerned people communicate caring; human caring is almost always helpful. Art is both enhanced and facilitated by practice. Artful communication is not a cautiously maneuvered discussion; yet the concepts and principles grasped are applied respectfully and intuitively. Intuition belongs more to an imaginative process than to formal learning: it is the ability to improve and perfect the use of knowledge from the depths of one's own experience and philosophy of life. Some persons are naturally perceptive. They have an innate ability for "reading others correctly," and for saying the right thing. Artful communication thus keeps the process from being artificial.

Science may free one from the limitations of personal experience and predilections; with science one seeks unbiased empirical evidence or formal validation of nursing hypotheses. Science can be used to increase the capacity to be helpful by enhancing innate abilities. The ability to be helpful can also be learned scientifically through the nursing process, which is a synthesis of emotions and intellect. The merger of emotions and knowledge may lead to insightful and creative communication patterns. Basic to the process of communication is the application of theoretical knowledge about human nature. Such theories, to be discussed later in more detail, aid in opening and keeping open the channels of communication. Principles can be learned, applied, and refined to the degree that the probability of reaching a desired outcome is increased. Mastery of scientific knowledge concerning human nature and the artful application of that which is learned is basic to the nursing process: an interdependent system of human activities and a scientific approach to solving human problems. In the discussion of the nursing process, Marriner's four descriptive steps, or phases, will be used.[12] The nursing process is a dynamic concept with change in the cyclic phases coinciding with change in the patient-care situation.

Assessment is the first phase of the nursing process. It is a systematic gathering of biopsychosocial data on the person to be helped. Knowledge of human behavior may help the nurse to know what to look for and what lines of inquiry to pursue and to analyze critically her observations and actions and their probable consequences. Commonalities with other patient-care situations and preconceived theoretical formulations are continuously checked against the presenting data: the patient's unique strengths, limitations, adaptive capacities, attitudes, and efforts to achieve health. What the nurse sees manifested is the interaction between a problem and a given personality. Because each person is different, every problem is different; so every time that the nurse assesses a patient with a problem, she sees a *different* problem and makes a different nursing diagnosis and preliminary plan of care.

The *planning* phase begins with the nursing diagnosis and involves the mutual participation of patient and nurse in the decision-making process. Through collaborative efforts, acceptable priorities and means to achieve short- and long-term ends, or goals, are defined. Goals represent a complex interaction between abilities and aspiration and are said to be more attainable when they are reasonable, measurable, and meaningful to the patient. Sometimes tentative-solution strategies must be based on a wide range of shifting behavioral signs and cues. The greater the knowledge and perceptivity of the nurse, the higher the level of inferences concerning the meaning of behavior and the predictive value concerning potential outcomes of her actions. Verifying a variety of inferences with the patient may preclude stereotyping if the significant findings are systematized into an individualized plan of care.

Implementation is the phase of deliberative nursing intervention. The nurse's conclusions are creatively and knowledgeably combined with the physician's orders in the actual giving of care. Continuous input from the patient, his family, and other care givers is coordinated and communicated in a written plan of care, so that the likelihood of achieving desired health results is maximized. The status of a person's health has a great deal to do with his feelings. The patient's mood, attitude, and reaction to the personal attributes of those caring for him influence the effectiveness of nursing care. Theoretical concepts concerning the nature of man may help the nurse to understand that *how* nursing care is done may be just as crucial as *what* is done. As in all other phases of the nursing process, human judgment is paramount in reassessing original hypotheses and making necessary care revisions. Judgment and knowledge work in concert, facilitating an awareness of and responsiveness to patients' problems and promoting favorable change along the health-illness continuum.

The final phase is *evaluation*. Naturally the patient and those intimately associated with him are part of this ongoing process, since the patient is the nurse's central concern. Evaluation helps to determine which problems were resolved and which require further deliberation. Knowledge of human nature may help to predict the consequences of nursing actions and to account for the success or failure of various approaches. Receptivity to feedback from all participants in the patient's care is essential in refining and developing innovative patterns of personalized care and in examining the efficacy of these actions.

The nursing process is involvement with another's personality. How the patient copes with tension and tears, handles anxiety and anger, deals with his own and another's sexuality, and expresses peace and pain are manifestations of his personality. Principles concerning man's personality have varying degrees of validity. Some concepts concerning basic human nature derive from the experience of trial and error; some are verified generalizations from specific helping situations; some are derived from common sense and some from research. Only through extensive use can their reliability be tested and their limitations recognized. The varying sources of principles give many choices of approaches and techniques. No one method is all things to all persons; therefore, not all interactions, or intervals in which the past experiences and expectations of patient and nurse mutually influence each other, require the same range of approaches and techniques. Some interactions are short; some are long. What is required, however, is the realization that all human interactions communicate something for good or ill. Communication is not limited to a fixed range of responses; it is highly variable and constantly changing. The nursing process is an opportunity-providing relationship for personal expressions of individuality and wholeness.

This does not presuppose that all individuals either need or want to ventilate, or air, their concerns in public. Some have marvelous inner and many outer resources: a support system of family and friends. Self-expression is not synonymous with self-disclosure. Patients have a right to engage in silent dialogue and to keep some thoughts private. Wolff questions the assumption that the sole purpose of nursing conversation is to help patients voice deep concerns that they cannot share with anyone else. Of course, this assumption has much validity when anxious moments and critical experiences are shared by those in close proximity, but, explains Wolff:

> By and large, patients are persons like you and me and are not completely lacking in human resources. Most have some trusted confidantes, close bonds of kinship or friendship or both. The large majority of people entering a hospital are not so devoid of human and spiritual sustenance that they have to look to the nurse as the *one* person to confide in, to sustain them, and see them through the inner turmoil which illness and its aftermath may cause.[13]

Thus communication principles, at times, are best applied when the nurse makes herself available by giving her presence and time. Some may make use of her presence; others may not.

Through the discriminate and conscious use of reason, the science of communication helps keep the process from being superficial. Communication in nursing that combines sensitivity (the art) with knowledge of human behavior (the science) views man holistically and, although it does not stay the onslaught of social paradoxes and pain, can

lessen their impact. The word *communication* has important deriva-
tions that are rarely mentioned in professional literature; the words are
to commune with. Nurses need to become more familiar with its meaning.

COMMUNICATION: THE CORE OF THE NURSE-PATIENT RELATIONSHIP
Description of relationship

In nursing as in many other professions the helping relationship is
described as being an "interpersonal one." To be more specific the singular terms of *nurse* and *patient* are hyphenated, so that they are made
compound. *Nurse-patient* suggests an intimate association between two
separate identities. This is not necessary. The very use of the term *interpersonal relationship* makes all else redundant. According to Webster,
in human relationships the word *interpersonal* means "existing between persons, relating or involving personal and social relationships
out of which develop . . . (1) . . . systems of shared expectations, (2) . . .
patterns of emotional relatedness, (3) . . . and modes of social adjustment."[14] Fortunately, such an all-encompassing definition could not be
the insignia of service for the nursing profession alone. Many allied
professionals, such as the clergy, counselors, social workers, teachers,
physical therapists, dieticians, and occupational therapists, can be consulted on behalf of the patient and his family. Inherent in the nursing
process is the synthesis of nursing activities with multidisciplinary activities.

However, nursing seems to have given this stated ideology more than
a temporary refuge. Nurses have rejoiced in the conception of this value
stance with perhaps too little thought of the complications that inhere
in the process of making a value viable!

Hall conceptualized three basic, interrelated components of the
nurse-patient relationship.[15] The first component is *nurturing,* which
correlates with caring and comforting and the intimate bodily care of
bathing, feeding, toileting, dressing, and moving. The second component—*curing*—is shared with the medical profession and helps the patient to make use of the physician's therapy in whatever ways the patient
successfully can. Curing is assisting the patient to cope with stressors
or stresses around or within that may lead to crises and irreversible
damage. The core of the nurse-patient relationship is the last component—*helping.* The focus is on interpersonal skills to help the individual
maximize all his potentials and achieve self-actualization. Similarly Peplau conceives of nursing as a significant interpersonal and therapeutic
process. The nurse collaborates with others "in organizing conditions
that facilitate forward movement of personality and other ongoing
human processes in the direction of creative, constructive, productive,

personal, and community living."[16] However, broad expanses can exist between consensus for an idea and its realization. Symbolic representations do not make interpersonal relationships; *words must come alive.*

The conflict and the division within the profession concerning the means to obtain ends may be a healthy sign of progress. Conflict is often a corollary to change, moving intellectual concepts to concrete implementations. Acknowledging current concern with nurse-patient relationships within the profession, Orlando states that "automatic inadequate communications between the patient and the nurse are what complicate the nurse-patient situation."[17] Therefore meaningful interpersonal relationships seem to depend on the quality of communication.

According to Mauksch and David,[18] nurses have yet to produce a visible, autonomously effective practice. The nursing process is identified as a means of unifying a profession now sadly divided, and its implementation is tantamount to survival. Current circumstances seem to lend considerable urgency to translating the "professional prose" of nursing philosophies into behavioral terms and collectively crystallizing purpose, process, and performance into effective communication patterns. Effective communication is central to interpersonal relationships and will help make sound the correspondence between idealism and reality.

From Webster's definition many human activities that are linked together by communication can be envisioned. The explanations of the deductions are part of Mauksch's and David's "Prescription for Survival" of the nursing profession.[18]

1. *Nursing is a social service.* The nursing process underlies nursing practice, the delivery of a broad, knowledge-based service designed to respond to societal needs. The needs are not qualified by physical, emotional, or social dysfunctions. The nursing process facilitates and reinforces the efforts of society toward health-sustaining behavior. Inherent in the process are the basic tenets of a discipline of service: accountability, scientific competence, peer review, and control over conditions of practice.

2. *There is direct contact with people.* The undisputed focus of the nursing process is human beings in one-to-one relationships. Goal development based on a comprehensive understanding of a person's needs and striving to meet these needs in a continuous and coordinated manner exemplifies a practice responding to a societal mandate.

3. *The contact is of a personal nature.* The nursing process is human endeavor. The nursing history, a systematic format for obtaining information about the person as a unique individual, replaces anomic approaches. The planning, implementation, and evaluation of care go

beyond task-oriented activities and involve attention to the exquisite details that make up human personalities.

4. *There is totality of involvement.* One of the motivating forces in the nursing process is reaching and touching the personal patterns of another's life experiences. Striving to know the meaning of the experience to the individual patient, the nurse must truly be with him and he with her. Both can better work together in alleviating the conditions that are mutually indentified as inhibiting valued change and growth. Without such involvement the nurse and the individual meet and part as strangers.

5. *The relationship is a shared one.* The individual usually experiences a community agency or institution through the person who provides the service. In many settings the benefits of an organization reach families through the nursing process. Together the nurse, the individual, his family, and other members of the health team exchange information and participate in making decisions. The patient's autonomy in making choices is supported maximally to the extent that his condition, circumstances, and competence permit.

6. *The relationship implies caring techniques.* Deep concern, regard, respect, and compassion may be communicated through the nursing process. Verbally and nonverbally the nurse translates these feelings and attitudes into intelligent and creative actions. Throughout the process, modest virtues, such as courtesy, find integral expression. Caring techniques involve emotions that are appropriately used to further the relationship.

7. *Life and limb are not necessarily being threatened.* The nursing process is a commitment to deliver service in accordance with the needs of the individual, whether they stem from the catastrophic ending of love or convalescence from a disease. Whatever the nature of the initial contact, the individual is offered help in mobilizing his own capacities to cope with the experience and to formulate objectives to meet his needs whenever feasible.

8. *The relationship involves feelings—the nurse's and others'.* The nursing process creates an atmosphere that fosters self-realization in the nurse and the individual. Each is freed from rigid, stereotyped behavior. "Freedom to be" promotes honest, direct, and uncontrived responses to what has been learned during the interaction. Learning may promote growth. Within the confines of ethics and judgment, the nurse gives of herself and is enriched by the giving. The individual, in turn, may communicate the kinds of things that would otherwise remain unknown: what he values, hopes, dreams or worries about, and feels. Feelings help to make the relationship personal; they help to individualize care.

9. *Knowledge of man is vital.* The nursing process uses the scientific method of problem solving and demonstrates nursing function through the synthesis and integration of humanity, art, science, and skills. This knowledge of mankind may help the nurse to explain the inexplicable balancing in one person of heredity, disease, character, temperament, and choice.

10. *One must learn to know oneself, as well as others.* The nursing process has as its basis a belief in the worth, uniqueness, dignity, and irreplaceability of each individual. The nurse must have self-awareness: a recognition of her flaws and foibles—her feelings and needs. If this part of her being is denied, the consequences may be a kind of self-alienation that devalues her own and another's human dimensions. To collaborate toward goals is extremely difficult if self-knowledge is excluded from human interactions, for honesty with another is subsequent to honesty with oneself.

Along with nursing, there are many configurations of helping relationships: doctor-patient, social worker–client, counselor-counselee, teacher-pupil, and parent-child, to name a few. That this acccepted pattern of word order places the persons in need of help in a subordinate role is no novel insight—no grammatical mishap. Admittedly the reasons for doing so are valid in some relationships. However, the apparent imperfections must be considered as they relate to nursing.

The helper gets "star billing." The one who by virtue of position sets the tone for what is to follow is the leader and is assumed to have knowledge, strength, wisdom, and expertise. Sometimes this is so; often it is not.

Implicit in the subordinate rank are also many conscious and unconscious value judgments that deny the dignity of man. The one being helped should be submissive, conforming, dependent, and grateful. If pursued to its logical conclusion, the condition is one of powerlessness. Although the helper-helpee relationship projects verbal symmetry on the surface, a true "being with" one another does not necessarily follow.

In the nursing profession the present continues to interact with the past. Some of the earliest nursing efforts were directed toward those who occupied an exceptionally low social position—those who demeaned the status of poverty with illness. The term *nurse-patient relationship* may have been an attempt to achieve status in a profession that could not confer status. Significant is nursing's heritage of the deep-seated mother image. The nurse was not an individual but a maternal surrogate: uneducated, intuitively wise, gentle, loving, kind, nurturing, indefatigable, and saintly. Such dedicated behavior was involved in a way of life that was little honored and rewarded. Nursing's symbolic mother image was aptly described by Peplau, who suggested that during the nurse-patient relationship, one of the nurse's functions is that of "psychological mothering: unconditional acceptance in a sustaining relationship that provides fully for need satisfaction" until the individual is able to meet his own needs adequately and independently.[19] However, patterns of relationships change; the perpetuation of the term *nurse-patient relationship* must be questioned.

It has been suggested that language is a forerunner of thought that affects behavior. "In the history of the individual, his language may well help to shape his picture of the world and influence his social actions."[20] If this is so, thought should be given to reordering the professional relationship to read *patient-nurse*. This is more than playing semantic games. *Patient-nurse relationship* will clearly focus priorities; by reshaping some of the nurse's thinking, it may better help her accomplish her goals. Precise thought precedes precise performance.

If this can be done, nurses will have grasped the connotative meaning of *interpersonal relationship*. This, more than the literal meaning of the words, will make for genuine contacts. Once the surface structure of a situation is set, it can be changed only as persons change. All are more comfortable in keeping unchanged the things that they have learned. The current word association of *nurse-patient* has a deep emotional component and a lulling quality. The usage of the term puts constraints on a relationship that nurses themselves have characterized as *dynamic*. *Patient-nurse* suggests a new way of responding throughout the phases of the nursing process. It puts the emphasis in all actions where it truly belongs and makes the relationship more equalitarian. Only then could the nurse belie Maslow's[21] conclusion that dominance-subordination patterns prevail because the dominant person attempts to gain security and self-esteem through control of another viewed as less adequate.

COMMUNICATION AND PERSONAL CHARACTERISTICS

Each participant may bring to a relationship helpful characteristics that are but expressions of desirable human traits. By no means do personal traits such as caring, trust, empathy, sympathy, respect, and humor exhaust the reservoir of desired human qualities; but such qualities of relatedness comprise a vital part of the nurse's professional vocabulary. *Rapport,* a particular way of perceiving and relating to our fellow human beings, *sums up* this cluster of helpful characteristics, which are inextricably tied up with the nurse's conception of human beings. Her personal biography—basic beliefs, attitudes, and feelings—largely determines her relationships with others. Rapport, in essence, transforms a series of nurse-patient contacts into meaningful patient-nurse relationships.[22] Rapport is the emotional matrix in which relationships are *established, maintained,* and *terminated.* Rapport is the matrix of emotional support—giving assistance, when indicated, compatible with the personal style of each patient and in the way in which the nurse is most comfortable. Rapport in the nursing process enables patients to cope with life experiences more and more through their own efforts.

Curiously enough, the idea somehow has been conveyed that cognition is contaminated by emotion. "Feeling" has been said to "get in the way"—but in the way of what? Feelings do not have to conflict with thinking. Normally they are complementary parts of the communication process. The epitome of true involvement is the intellect tempered by emotions. Feelings get in the way only when one is either overwhelmed or "underwhelmed" by them: when one's perceptual field is distorted to the detriment of the patient.

Communication is catalyzed by caring, trust, empathy, sympathy, respect, and humor. These traits channeled into thought can convey in ways that are useful, expressions of tenderness and deep sensitivity through nursing techniques. Moreover, these personal characteristics are not mutually exclusive. They may overlay and fuse with the nursing process. They function well when finely balanced, highly personalized, properly timed, and precisely focused. Note that these characteristics do not meet the requirements of a situation demanding certainty.

Trying to explain what each personal trait is meant to accomplish is a delicate matter. Many terms have become interchangeable. For example, one can read about *openness* and find a discussion of *genuineness.* One could look up *authenticity* and find a description of *congruence.* Still, a certain amount of self-disclosure on the part of nurses and patients is essential to effective communication. Emphasis is placed on the fact that nurses' actions need to be consistent with their words. Hypocrisy has no place in the nursing process. As an instance, if one says "good morning" to a patient who comes to the nurses' station, this salutation should not convey the message, "Oh, no! Here's that pest again! What a way to start the day!"

Caring

In nursing the interpersonal relationship is a caring one. Caring is akin to warmth. It differs from warmth in that it is more enduring and more unconditional. Caring comes from a reverence for life; this general appreciation of humanity translates into concern for the cares of the individual. Caring creates a social climate that communicates feelings of goodwill and concern when feelings cannot be put into words. Human pain has many sources: the physical diseases that scourge man, as well as wounds of the mind and spirit. The challenge is to learn that cure of the patient is inseparable from *caring* for him.

Nurses know what they do when in the strict sense they are giving care. More importantly people know how they feel when they are "cared for." These are value judgments; giving and receiving care mean different things to each individual. The nurse may think that she has given good care if her patient did as much for himself as possible during the morning bath and offered no complaints. On the other hand, the patient might have felt better cared for if he had been allowed to sleep. Needless to say the relationship would have been enhanced for both had there been more fellowship of feelings.

Caring is careful listening. It communicates a sense of worth: what the patient says is "worthwhile, worth understanding, and that consequently *he* is worthwhile for having said it. . . ."[23] Caring is the voluntary communication of love. It is investing some of yourself in the patient, sharing a part of life together, participating in the problems presented in the recovery from illness or in preventing an illness from occurring, and sharing part of a family's grief when death occurs or the happiness of a little boy when you tell him that he no longer needs to have injections.[24] Caring communicates a tenderness for the self known as *self-respect,* or *dignity.* To be tender is to care; to be tender is to be soft and vulnerable and to risk pain. Human caring is compassion for another. "Its biological roots lie in the maternal and paternal behavior of all higher living things; and it is reinforced by environmental circumstances. *Most important of these is the presence of caring in another human being.*" Upon it rests survival.[25]

Another risk in caring is that it can be misinterpreted and emotionally entangle the nurse and the patient in threatening situations if the purpose of the relationship is not clear to both participants. Compassion is not romantic involvement; compassion must contribute to the goals of the patient-nurse relationship. The pain of previous involvement in unsatisfactory relationships may make the patient wary. The relationship must first be tested for truth and constancy before he feels safe enough to risk interpersonal closeness with the nurse. Caring involves a sense of proportion, not an invasion of privacy. This is not to say that nurses must constantly adjust their "thermostats of warmth" to highs and lows, but rather be alert to possible consequences when adjustments are not made.

Trust

The nurse can create a context in which an interpersonal relationship can commence but cannot by herself bring it into being. A commonality to all successful interpersonal beginnings is trust, without which a relationship becomes emotionally impoverished and stagnant.

Trust is "a sensing, a feeling, that at least some important sectors of the world are dependable, and that some of the people in the world are warm, caring, available, and friendly."[26] Through the nursing process the nurse's trust and confidence in the profession are conveyed. One cannot discuss trust without speaking of honesty. The patient can entrust himself to the care of others only if he honestly has confidence in them. This presumes that patients must have faith in what nurses say and do if the relationship is to develop into a trusting one. Consequently, it is most desirable that the nurse and patient perceive each other as being trustworthy during the *initial phase* of the relationship because who would reveal himself to someone felt to be not "for him?" The nurse believes that the patient is being honest; similarly the patient believes that the nurse is being honest. Since behavior often begets its own kind, this shared belief helps to establish and maintain a mutually trusting interpersonal relationship.

Emotional and physical helplessness impose dependency. The patient must trust others to do what he cannot do for himself. This makes for feelings of insecurity—of being unsafe. Each step forward in the relationship is made possible by honesty, which decreases his sense of personal vulnerability. Feelings of being safe allow for retreat when necessary. Nurses will be with him in favorable and unfavorable circumstances. Once the patient perceives that he is "in good hands," he may communicate more about his true self. As a result of this communication the relationship is more likely to be maximally helpful.

Notice furthermore that mutual trust is said to be sustained by an honest sharing of information—that honesty in patients calls forth honesty in nurses. However, many gray areas come to mind. Honesty may not be delimited by positive or negative responses. It could lie somewhere in between, since nurses know much that is not to be shared with patients. Sometimes it is the patient's prognosis; more often it is the patient's diagnosis. Traditionally these two areas are thought to be within the physician's province. Still, at times, nurses are instructed to explore the patient's diagnosis with him. With the diabetic patient the diagnosis is discussed in much detail and must be done so repeatedly if the patient is to participate therapeutically in his plan of care, but such is not always the case, particularly when the illness is terminal.

Another inconsistency concerns patients' prognoses. Few, if any, constraints are placed on informing patients of a good prognosis. Such news can be readily communicated. Conversely, patients with poor prognoses may have difficulty in obtaining honest answers. What is more likely to be communicated is false optimism that causes feelings of disillusionment and mistrust. In a different sense a patient may ask the nurse if the surgeon is competent. The nurse's experience may lead her to question the physician's competence. A response on her part mandates a clear choice between loyalty and slander. Many imponderables in mutual trust admit of no easy solutions.

Guidelines may be all that one can offer for dubious situations. Inherent in a relationship of mutual trust is the right of both participants to say no. Nurses need to admit that they cannot answer some questions. At the same time the nurse should be ever alert to the question with hidden meaning. Nurses should not ignore questions. Clearly their responsibility is to inform the patient that with his permission the question will be referred to a person who is more qualified to respond. Nurses may feel that it is in the best interest of the patient to have his questions answered honestly. Implicit in this belief, however, is the nurse's recognition of and willingness to assume *responsibility* for the patient's reaction. To be responsible is to be "accountable, to be answerable for something, to be liable, to be able to satisfy any reasonable claim involving important work or trust; a duty; a charge."[27] Honesty, like all the other general helping traits, is not operant on all-or-none laws.

Empathy

What is there about empathy that gains it so many adherents? First, empathy is a type of intellectual role playing, an attempt to experience the emotional state of an individual *as if* one were in his place. Rogers[28] describes the state of being empathetic as perceiving "the internal frame of reference" of another with accuracy—to perceive the patient "himself as he is seen by himself"—to sense his hurt or pleasure as he senses it but without losing the *as if* condition. Nurses, by conscious effort, may gain a glimpse of the patient's "in-there" world and see the "out-there" world *as if* through the patient's eyes. Hopefully nurses can achieve oneness with the patient's world to such a degree that it is their world for a time. The way the world appears to one person is different from the way it appears to another. Although the external world may seem the same, the "internal" world is each individual's subjective assessment. Certainly beauty is in the eye of the beholder.

Not surprisingly, the individual's internal vision of the world may blind him psychologically to objective reality and lead to misconceptions. Each person's reality can be skillfully handled by perceptual attitudes and personal outlooks: imagination, conflicts, wishes, and feelings. Each person responds differently to life's situations, and each behaves differently within the same setting. Viewing the individual from his own internal frame of reference and concentrating on *his experience* of reality can facilitate the nursing process. Once the meaning of an experience is clarified, it may be dealt with and the emotional impact shared.

Like an actor in a play, one can submerge oneself in a role; yet psychologically one does not become the character to remain so forever but resumes one's own identity once the play is ended. The identification is temporary. A corollary example is the feeling experienced when one reads a good book or sees a play or movie. So engrossed does one become that one "cannot put the book down" or becomes figuratively glued to the seat. So closely can one identify with characters that mood, attitudes, and points of view of others are more easily understood. Good books and good plays are said to have something for everyone. The inference is made that, in relation to nursing, such a vicarious perception of another's world leads to a better understanding of his behavior. The patient may be better helped to cope with the symptoms that he is manifesting.

Empathy is said to result when one has walked awhile in another's shoes. Only by attempting to take the patient's place can the nurse experience his internal frame of reference. Since no one can truly enter the subjective world of another, the shoes will not be a snug fit, but the journey will not be for naught. Such involvement can help nurses see patients in terms of what they are and not what they "ought" to be. At the end of the journey the nurse should consciously be more appreciative of the feelings of others.

Another parallel is the fact that empathy is a personalized type of communication wherein the nurse tries to tune directly into another's wavelength. Objectivity is required to prevent the nurse's own values from distorting the message. In general, having similar experiences facilitates tuning in on another's wavelength. This may explain the deeper understanding that some parents have for other parents. However, achieving harmony is more difficult if there is social distance because of differences in age, sex, status, race, and culture. Most people have a natural tendency to edit communication according to their own unique patterns of experience and customary ways of thinking.

In conclusion, empathy is a type of cognition that should lead to a broader scope of nursing care. It is a specific type of data gathering preparatory to taking action. This perception of patient's problems should better help nurses contemplate what to do. Unless successfully communicated to patients, empathy may become apathy. Patients who look for understanding are sensitive to even the slightest signs of disinterest or disapproval. Therefore patients must sense through the nurse's behavior that they are understood. Empathy should be, but is not necessarily, "active" understanding. Empathy may have a special attraction for professionals because the degree of emotional involvement is prescribed. Empathy has an *"as if"* quality; the personal risks are thus not too great. It is an essentially neutral process and does not necessarily mean that the nurse uses her comprehension for nursing activities.

Sympathy

Adler defined sympathy as being "the purest expression of social feelings. Whenever we find sympathy in a human being, we can in general be sure that his social feeling is mature, because this affect allows us to judge how far a human being is able to identify with his fellow men."[29] Sympathy is a socially sanctioned behavior, a fusion of feeling with action. We communicate sympathy at times of deep hurt to help alleviate the pain of mental or physical suffering. At such times a common reaction is to "offer one's sympathy." Another's distress is felt, and we, in turn, respond by giving something of ourselves in offering comfort. Still, to want to relieve another's distress does not mean that this can always tangibly be done. Nevertheless, sympathy conveys both the desire and the compassion felt in failure. The patient understands; because he has one's sympathy, he knows that he matters. His sorrows will be eased through others' support and encouragement.

Sympathy is one of the humanizing qualities of rapport—a specific expression of compassion, warmth, kindness, interest, and concern.[30] This caring quality that urges one to action cannot be feigned despite the most elaborate communication techniques. Such attitudes, types of thinking, and feelings are the heart of the nursing process.

However, in nursing, sympathy is suspect—somehow not in keeping with the professional image. Nurses should be of stout heart. In the nurse, sympathy is seen as a loss of control that facilitates or maintains a similar loss in the patient. Images wherein both the nurse and patient are reduced to a state of hysterical immobilization are conjured up. The assumption is made that once a patient has had an encounter with sympathy it will be so gratifying that he will never again be the same: all his subsequent behaviors will be directed toward gaining more sympathy. This will have a negative cumulative effect: the more sympathy he gains, the more dependent he will become. Such unbridled self-indulgence will lead to irreparable harm.

In reality, little danger exists that nurses will become a source of need gratification in response to patients' emotional outpourings. Much maudlin behavior, moreover, would not necessarily increase his dependence. Satisfaction of a need should decrease its intensity or cause it to disappear. Instead of the patient's becoming more dependent, he should become more responsible. Therefore an expression of sorrow by the nurse need not encourage sorrow in the patient. Instead, sympathy can serve as a helpful approach: an offer to share some of the patient's problems at a time when he cannot manage them alone. The snowballing effect is that the patient gains strength from this mutual sharing and becomes more, instead of less, able to solve problems.

Somewhere in between a sympathetic and an unsympathetic feeling lies pity, which is something of a taboo in nursing. It is a feeling that should be reserved for *oneself alone: a warm and natural concern* when things go wrong in our world. To feel sorry for oneself is perfectly all right. However, to feel sorry for others may be wrong.

Saying "you poor thing" is not ipso facto a sign of contempt, and it does not mean that a person is seen as an object. Consider the many variations of the following incident. A child falls while running and bruises himself. His mother helps him up and while holding him close soothes him by saying, "Oh, you poor thing. Show me where it hurts. I'll kiss it and make it well." This approach is much more therapeutic than the stiff-upper-lip admonishment, "Big boys don't cry." There is warmth and humanness in the first interaction. The mother does not relate to the child as a "thing"; the child does not respond as a thing. Once comforted, children usually show their natural propensity for challenging the world again and risking another collision with an immovable object. This brief example is designed to show that no communication that conveys true concern for another should be repudiated outright. Even though pity is a fleeting and rather unreliable emotion, it can sustain some persons even if only for a brief span of time. Again note that techniques must be adapted to each unique relationship.

In this culture the virtue of independence is so exalted that those who may be less self-reliant are too easy to view with disdain. However, there are times in all our lives when we are dependent and need time to marshall our resources. Allowing this time is not a patronizing type of "giving" to someone who "loves misery." Sympathy, an active involvement with another, should become a part of the social contract in the nursing process. "When a nurse sympathizes with a patient, she communicates to him that she wants to assist him, is concerned about him—not because he is Bed 19 and she is expected to give nursing care, but because he is himself and no one else."[30]

Respect

Nurses see many persons who are vastly different than they. This obvious conclusion hardly enchants the intellect with an erudite or original thought. In this society one tends to focus on visible differences and take these distinctions as valid measures of those scrutinized. The result is very little reflection on the question: "What is there about man that thou art mindful of him?" Just saying that people are different is superfluous if one disregards the most basic of all human differences —human emotional responses. Both the patient and the nurse are never free from the inward authority of subjective needs, values, beliefs, attitudes, and motives that have been integrated into their cognitive systems. Previous learning and experience are more meaningful than biologic makeup and cause each person to be certain that the mosaic of life he builds slowly, painfully, and piece by piece is the true one. Man craves certainty and communicates through a sociocultural network of preferences and prejudices that gives consistency and continuity to his life; yet relativity of meaning is now applicable to what was once adamantly proposed to be a physically stable universe.

Distinctive ways of handling reality may enable individuals to function well within their own groups but handicap, rather than help, communication when each participant's culturally conditioned view of the world radically differs. Differences in cultural patterning may create conflict between the norms and health values of the patient and nurse. With ease we can identify others' unreasonable ways while remaining oblivious to the way in which we seem unreasonable to them. Since much of our learning comes from traditional thought, we seldom consider the fact that the way we *see* the world is not the way the world actually *is* but simply what we were taught about it. Respect includes mindfulness of the differences in man's cognitive systems; and, although these may cause friction, respect involves resisting the temptation to recruit others to one's personal versions of reality. Respect recognizes that one's personal memoirs are part of one's intrinsic worth.

To communicate respect is hard work. It means in essence that the nurse must transcend her own culture to have a magnified, rather than myopic, view of man. Respect is easier to give those whose belief systems mirror one's own. Presumably it is easier for the nurse to communicate with a patient holding compatible views because both are speaking the same language. For clarification I must point out that much of one's vocabulary consists of antonyms to facilitate a classification of flora, fauna, and folk. A trend to forsake is the kind of categorizing that ignores the qualities that make individuals unique and deals only in those qualities believed to be shared. The real self becomes indistinguishable from stereotypes when man is dichotomized as good-bad, deserving-undeserving, and important-unimportant. Seeing the patient in terms of "should be" rather than "now is" ignores the rich qualities that give relationships their human quotients. One implication of respect is seeing each patient with complete freshness, instead of relying on familiar but often fictitious images. Respect includes valuing another whose "social value" may not be visible.[31]

Implicit in respect is the concept of acceptance of man in his totality: what he is and what he does; yet behavior that results from a patient's perceptions has a reality impact ethically, morally, and legally. Thus *total* acceptance seems to be a difficult conceptual stance to take. Total acceptance of *all* behavior implies that the patient is able to control himself within the context of the situation. This is especially true if one thinks of the limits that must be set at times to keep the patient from harming himself or others. To say that, although the nurse accepts the existence of the patient's needs that motivate behavior, the behavior itself may be unacceptable is not a contradiction; *but* it is not judged as making the patient less worthy. The nurse cannot always fulfill or allow the patient to fulfill his needs. The patient, however, should not be condemned for having them.

An innocent way of stating the aforementioned concept is to examine the following: A basic axiom of child rearing is that parents while approving of the child can at the same time be disapproving of his behavior. Moreover, they should make this difference apparent in disciplining the child; that is, the parent is not chastising him per se, but his behavior. The distinction is not easy for either the parents or the child.

To go a step further, another misunderstanding about respect is a belief in the necessity for automatic and mutual liking. This places unreasonable demands on both patients and nurses. Liking may come, but also it may not. Should it develop, it represents a bonus; but all successful performances are not so favorably rewarded. Although for patients to dislike nurses who are doing everything possible to help is difficult, such a result is not impossible. Dislike may be mutual; the patient and the nurse may perceive each other to be threatening. Threats occur in situations incongruent with one's favored self-conception, responses, and relationships. Defensive behavior is mobilized to protect one's personal frame of reference. Having recognized her dislike of the patient, the nurse must take care not to translate her feelings into actions. Remember that the more inner security one has, the less likely one is to feel threatened by or be threatening to others.

Despite the nurse's knowledge of the cultural dimensions of human beings and the appropriate application of this knowledge, she and a particular patient may be unable to work effectively toward goals in a specific situation. Pretense—self-alienation to win approval—has no place in the nursing process. Differences do not disappear because they are denied, and a patient's right to help is not synonymous with his readiness to receive help. We can command attention by making people stop and look but cannot make them listen to our messages and understand our meanings. This does not mean that the patient-nurse relationship has no value. Value is found in learning that unjustified criticism and rejection is a risk in all human relationships. Communication accomplishes its purpose if the message is interpreted by the patient and the nurse with *respect* for disagreements concerning the content.

Humor

Life is neither all tragedy nor all comedy but strangely mixed. Most persons experience varying proportions of each. Humor is essential to good mental health. The solemnities of life need not preoccupy those involved in an interpersonal relationship. The nurse should strive for a balance between humor and solemnity.

Of all the emotional traits, humor is the most visible. Smiles and laughter draw attention. Who has a "sense of it" and who has not is usually easy to tell. Furthermore, humor is a familiar pattern of communication that people encounter in their everyday lives. Persons who have appropriately good humor are said to be easier to converse with. In contrast, to say that a person has a poor sense of humor or none at all is a reproach, implying the ability to see only the dreary side of life. Worse yet is to be described as "out of humor" or constantly morose. Everyone tries to give people a wide berth when they are in a bad mood.

Humor is like a handshake. It is one way to establish a warm interpersonal relationship rather quickly. Social distance is decreased, since laughter comes only if the persons involved are of like minds. Humor, a social bond, helps to break the ice between strangers. Admission to the hospital can be a frightening experience. To some the hospital is a threatening milieu with many unknowns. One spry old lady who was experiencing severe pain from a fractured hip proclaimed to the physician and nurse in attendance that she didn't want any special favors; they should just treat her as they would any other patient of noble birth. This affirmation of dignity set a tone of warmth for the relationship that grew in consideration of one for the other. Humor may have increased the physician's and nurse's awareness of the patient's individuality, discomfort, and unease. Such understanding can be beneficial by bringing people together.

Perhaps humor is an effective technique in communication because it suggests that the respondent is natural and unaffected. In this regard, humor has childlike qualities of playfulness. If one can be playful, one still has vestiges of youth and vigor. When one ceases to have such youthful relish, one is rigid, old, and infirm. So the old man is proud of his playful jokes that assure him that, arthritic as are his joints, he is a part of the mainstream. Thus the wheelchair becomes his "Cadillac" that is "parked" at night by his bed. A further implication is that to be humorous is to be momentarily free. He can disregard the inconvenience—the cares and woes of blinding necessity that occupy most of his time. Rather than succumb to his limitations, he can be amused by them. Humor, a defense mechanism, mentally modifies stressful situations and helps one to cope.

Humor helps to ease our passage through awkward moments. To make light of a matter is to distract. An incident can be brought to amusing conspicuousness. Laughter, instead of condemnation, will follow if both persons are "good sports" and can "take a joke." At times the blunder can be explained with a logic or illogic of one's own that can be more placating than an outright apology. For example, a student nurse was analyzing a urine specimen in the presence of an instructor; while pouring the specimen from the container into the test tube, the student accidentally dropped the container, splattering the contents on both their shoes and stockings. Somewhat alarmed by what had transpired, the student blurted out, "You can always depend on me to give you the benefit of the dirt." This humorous interpretation made the incident acceptable to the instructor and helped the student manage her anxiety.

Humor has a "merciful" aspect that gives patients a sense of triumph over adversity. This personal characteristic may have a function in preserving the sense of self. Humor may be an expression of the patient's unique capacity to adapt through denial by trying to avoid painful feelings from the impact of constantly confronting his illness. Humorous get-well cards help him to do this. Highly ritualized, impersonal hospital routines and authoritarian figures are made ridiculous and intrusive procedures hilarious. The cards imply that the recipient is only temporarily "out of action" and in no real danger: all is well. Fears seem less justified when one can jest about them. Laughter helps release anxiety in a conventional manner and puts distance between oneself and the problem. When inner security is eroding, humor is a classic means of conserving human hope; but humor falls flat when anxiety is overwhelming.

Humor can also serve as an outlet for a grievance: a gripe is disguised in an amusing form so as not to offend. A direct complaint carries the real or imagined threat of retaliation. One patient told a nurse after she hurriedly put him on a stretcher, so that he would not be late in being x-rayed, that the thing he admired most about her was her "sainted patience!" Through a jocular aside the patient made known his justifiable irritation.

Humor can wound. Vindictive practical jokes, such as giving someone a broken chair to sit in and laughing at the mishap, have the component of aggressive motivation. Lorenz, noting the association between humor, hostility, and aggression, explains that laughter, the overt expression of humor, can be used " . . . like aggressive dogs . . . set on and made to attack practically any enemy that reason may choose."[32] Humor is a cruel weapon that injures when one's laughter hurts another. Children are especially defenseless; to laugh at or make fun of a child is inexcusable. Humor is unhealthy when it leads to a pathologic denial of reality. Perennial show-offs or cutups, who do not stop long enough to admit or to express their true feelings, fall into this category.[33]

Nonsense does not mean no sense; humor can convey messages that edify, reassure, and release anxiety, as well as entertain. Light banter has a place in interpersonal relationships, and canned laughter from the radio and television need not be the only sounds of mirth that are heard. The primary usefulness of humor in a situation is the serving of needs; the type, technique, or content of humor is less important. Humor is healthy when it draws persons closer together in the immediate situation and helps individuals to handle reality.[33] At times it is "the best medicine."

TERMINATING THE PATIENT-NURSE RELATIONSHIP

The same patterns of relatedness that the nurse uses in establishing and maintaining a therapeutic alliance are helpful in bringing the relationship to a satisfactory conclusion. Caring, trust, empathy, sympathy, respect, and humor may help the nurse to subordinate her therapeutic ambitions to the patient's wishes and encourage what he can accomplish in a reasonable time interval. Prolonged contact or premature termination may respectively reflect the nurse's need to have a particular patient dependent on her or to foster independence without due regard for patient readiness. Ideally the mutuality of the decision to terminate is part of the initial goal-setting process. Information concerning roles and the times that the nurse and patient will be working together is exchanged and priorities set. Specific time limits may increase the impetus or the tempo of the working alliance. Knowing what to expect in the relationship helps each to determine the extent of involvement and allows for sufficient time to deal with feelings about separation.

During the relationship the nurse and patient may have shared much that is meaningful and intimate. Consequently, attitudes of attachment that are difficult to contend with may be present. In the process of separation a sense of loss, helplessness, loneliness, and grief makes parting difficult.[34] Termination can be emotional, and with sensitivity and timing it should be discussed periodically when feelings are neither high nor low.

The definition of the interpersonal relationship makes mention of the fact that the person is helped to "develop modes of social adjustment." In this regard the centrality of rapport in the communication may enhance the patient's ability to reach out and form other satisfying relationships in the community. Whether the patient's problems were resolved, mitigated, or made tolerable, the mutual evaluation of the experience in an atmosphere of rapport may reinforce the therapeutic outcome. The patient's lament, "The nurse never said a word about leaving," has a tone of reproach and abandonment. The patient feels rejected and hurt; whatever gains were made in the relationship, as well as the projections for aftercare, may be lost or disregarded. Then too the likelihood exists that feelings of disappointment may be transferred to another helper and make "mutual trust," if not an abstraction, very difficult.

A therapeutic relationship does not result in finished products. The process of growth continues in both nurses and patients. A relationship that has helped one to appreciate the value of another leads to increased feelings of self-worth. This higher self-esteem in both patient and nurse will serve them well in coping with the vagaries of life, even though they no longer are together. The significance of the termination phase in the patient-nurse relationship should be more formally recognized.

THE NURSE AS HELPER

Nurses, like patients, are unique individuals. They have their own thoughts, feelings, customs, attitudes, needs, desires, and reactions that are communicated to others. Little, if any, of their sociocultural background, education, state of health, life experiences, and self-concept will be left outside the patient's unit. To put the matter rather succinctly, nurses are not "neutral beings." Like other people, nurses are thinking and feeling all the time; so any notion of their making value-free assessments is somewhat of an illusion. Yet much of worth is found in the admonishment to be nonjudgmental. In the nursing process the nonjudgmental nurse does not speak or act as a critic of human affairs. She accepts the fact that, in spite of certain fundamental similarities, human beings are markedly different. She refrains from urging, advising, exhorting, and persuading her patient to change his interpersonal behavior so that she can function more comfortably in the relationship. She uses praise judiciously, since praise is but approval of behavior that is personally valued. The nonjudgmental nurse puts distance between first impressions and conclusions by jointly gathering, assessing, and evaluating data with the patient. Nonjudgmental approaches allow for exceptions and amendments: a receptivity to new knowledge.

The "self" is only therapeutic when one is conscious of it. This type of self-consciousness, or self-awareness, includes neither morbid introspection nor the kind of preoccupation that might lead to embarrassed and inhibited behavior. Consciousness of self equates with an awareness of one's strengths and weaknesses, capabilities and liabilities, and prejudices and preferences. This way of regarding self will help one gain a better perspective that leads to confidence. Self-confidence permits one to be more open, authentic, and genuine when interacting with others. Moreover, integrity usually follows from such an honest appraisal of self.

The nurse who is aware of the breadth and depth of her own real self can better relate to her patients and encourage, or at least not block communication. On the other hand, suppression of the real self leads to cool and contrived mannerisms, which desensitize the nurse to her own experiences and lead to impersonal contacts, rather than interpersonal relationships.[35]

With effective communication one may, without mythic exaggeration, turn most encounters into meaningful human interactions. An idea remains inert; concepts and principles remain views; and realities remain but possibilities without communication, for communication is essential to implementation. Communication is the chief means of matching nursing expertise to patients' problems.

The nurse can individualize care: communication is the essence of one-to-one relationships. The nurse can be creative—can integrate her knowledge of human behavior for novel and inventive approaches, develop her own style, and free herself from stereotyped and conventional clichéd responses. Joy is possible! Communication enriches: entrance to the perceptual world of another leads to a type of self-discovery that increases the ability to solve one's own problems. This type of problem solving is a valuable asset when untried abilities are put to the test.

Nursing of the past has no future! If nurses are contented with the status quo and if they fail to find new and better ways to deliver health care, "the reality of future nursing will be that of the epitaph."[36] *Change* is the only permanent aspect of any social contract. Effective communication is the key to changing nursing today and unlocking doors in nursing tomorrow.

REFERENCES

1. Henderson, V.: The nature of nursing, American Journal of Nursing **64**:62-68, 1964.
2. Smith, D.: Change: how shall we respond to it? Nursing Forum **4**:391-399, 1970.
3. Kramer, M.: Reality shock: why nurses leave nursing, St. Louis, 1974, The C. V. Mosby Co., p. 4.
4. Ibid., p. 23.
5. Ibid., p. 13.
6. Barnett, K.: A theoretical of the concepts of touch in nursing, Nursing Research **21**:102-110, 1972.
7. Krieger, D.: Therapeutic touch: the imprimatur of nursing, American Journal of Nursing **75**:784-787, 1975.
8. Skipper, J., Mauksch, H., and Tagliacozzo, D.: Some barriers to communication, Nursing Forum **2**:14-23, 1963.
9. Spitz, R.: Hospitalism, Psychoanalytic Study of the Child **1**:53-74, 1945.
10. The world book dictionary, vol. 1, Chicago, 1970, Field Enterprises Educational Corporation, p. 1268.
11. Toffler, A.: Future shock, New York, 1970, Random House, Inc., p. 149.
12. Marriner, A.: The nursing process: a scientific approach to nursing care, St. Louis, 1975, The C. V. Mosby Co., pp. 1-4.
13. Wolff, I.: The educated heart, American Journal of Nursing **63**:58-60, 1965.
14. Webster's third new international dictionary, Springfield, Mass., 1971, G. & C. Merriam Co., Publishers, p. 1181.
15. Bowar-Ferres, S.: Loeb Center and its philosophy of nursing, American Journal of Nursing **75**:810-815, 1975.
16. Peplau, H.: Interpersonal relations in nursing: a conceptual frame of reference for psychodynamic nursing, New York, 1952, G. P. Putnam's Sons, p. 12.
17. Orlando, I.: The dynamic nurse-patient relationship, New York, 1961, G. P. Putnam's Sons, pp. 69-70.

18. Mauksch, G., and David, M.: Prescription for survival, American Journal of Nursing **72:**2189-2193, 1972.
19. Peplau, op. cit., p. 40.
20. Krech, D., Crutchfield, R., and Ballachey, E.: Individual in society; a textbook of social psychology, New York, 1962, McGraw-Hill Book Co., p. 303.
21. Maslow, A.: Self-esteem, dominance feeling and sexuality in women, Journal of Social Psychology **16:**259-294, 1942.
22. Travelbee, J.: What do we mean by rapport? American Journal of Nursing **63:**70-72, 1963.
23. Rogers, C.: Carl Rogers describes his way of facilitating encounter groups, American Journal of Nursing **71:**276, 1971.
24. Macdonald, B.: Nursing's many meanings, American Journal of Nursing **14:**56-57, 1966.
25. Sobel, D.: Human caring, American Journal of Nursing **69:**2612-2613, 1969.
26. Poland, R.: Human experience: a psychology of growth, St. Louis, 1974, The C. V. Mosby Co., p. 17.
27. Fagin, C.: Nurse's rights, American Journal of Nursing **75:**82-85, 1975.
28. Rogers, C.: Client-centered therapy, Boston, 1951, Houghton Mifflin Co., p. 29.
29. Adler, A.: Understanding human nature, London, 1962, George Allen & Unwin, Ltd., pp. 276-277.
30. Travelbee, J.: What's wrong with sympathy? American Journal of Nursing **64:**68-71, 1964.
31. Wolff, op. cit., p. 39.
32. Lorenz, C.: On aggression, New York, 1963, Harcourt Brace Jovanovich, Inc., p. 285.
33. Robinson, V.: Humor in nursing, American Journal of Nursing **70:**1065-1069, 1970.
34. Hale, S., and Richardson, J.: Terminating the nurse-patient relationship, American Journal of Nursing **60:**63-66, 1960.
35. Jourard, S.: The bedside manner, American Journal of Nursing **60:**63-66, 1970.
36. Bennett, L.: This I believe: that nursing may become extinct, Nursing Outlook **18:**28-32, 1970.

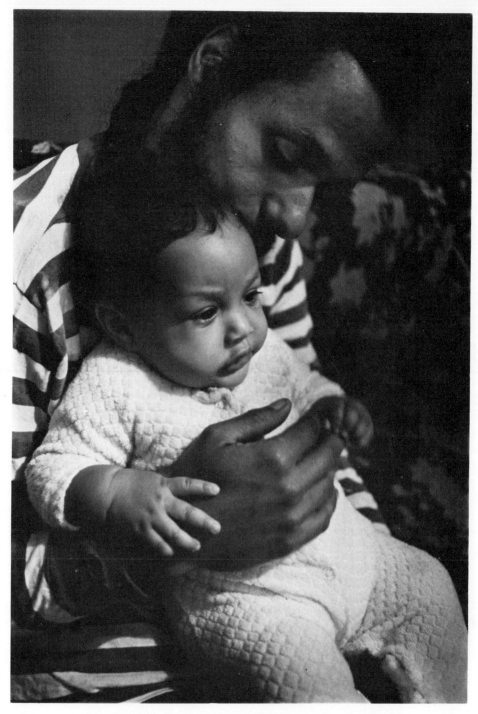

Man is a biologic organism . . . characterized by a life cycle and a capacity to develop in many ways. All his behavior has meaning and is multidetermined. From intimate experiences with others, he develops an identity, ideals, and expectations concerning his life and life roles. Intimate associations seem necessary for emergence of the best self—the most rational self—for a satisfying existence in society today. (Photograph by James Carroll, Editorial Photocolor Archives.)

CHAPTER 2

Theoretical assumptions concerning the nature of human beings

OVERVIEW

Many theories, or explanatory proposals, have been advanced to explain human behavior. Having an appreciation of theoretical possibilities is inseparable from having a deep appreciation of human beings. Nurses need to understand human behavior because communication itself is but a system of human interaction.

Theoretical assumptions are working hypotheses that often take the exceptions to prove the rule. For example, individuals must take in oxygen to live, whether the process of respiration is natural or artificial. Nothing in our experience indicates otherwise. Hence there is no description of an anaerobic human. Since this phenomenon is all-pervasive, there is no need to subject it to scientific inquiry and formulate the theorem that *Homo sapiens* sustains life by taking in oxygen. It would have no relevance. It is a part of our daily experience of which we are not even conscious unless the process becomes impaired. We all share the same frame of reference, since there are no outlines on this universal background of sameness.

However, should we encounter an exceptional person or two who survive by taking in carbon dioxide, our frame of reference would need critical reappraisal. A rule or norm concerning oxygen intake would then be in order to explain either the constancy of occurrence of oxygen breathers or the contradiction of finding carbon dioxide breathers.

So it was with Freud, who related hysterical patterns of behavior to the assumption that unconscious motivations determine actions. If all people exhibited hysterical behavior without exception, including Freud himself, there would be no need for theories explaining the phenomenon of hysteria. In other words, Freud did not need to attempt to give reasons for the basic consistencies that he observed in human behavior. Thus theories can help one to account for a kaleidoscope of observable human responses, both similar and different.

RELATIONSHIP OF BEHAVIORAL THEORIES TO COMMUNICATION

People are gatherers and processors of information. They store up their pasts, as well as much of their present and future potentials. Being social animals, they must communicate some of this data to others by audible word or silent gesture. In this sharing the first law of nature, preservation of self, will be operant; man tends to adopt a variety of maneuvers to prevent revelations that might lower self-esteem. To see this is to expect perversities in behavior as almost routine. The only antidote is thoughtful consideration of theoretical concepts that hold strategic suggestions for understanding the causes of human behavior, as well as the predictability of some behaviors.

Thoughtful consideration of any one theory may support the following conclusions: Theories are cognitive guidelines, directing the way and clearing the path to understanding. In offering a whole spectrum of possibilities for the exploration of infinite human variety, theories represent some of the surest avenues available to effective interactions. For better exercise of judgment these informed assumptions cause one to pause and reconsider familiar forms of thoughts and reactions before going ahead. These guidelines suggest what to look for in communication and how to systematically make sense of what is communicated. Theories lead to a scrutiny of our observations and as a consequence the selection of a better choice of means to accomplish ends. In summary, each guideline helps one see more clearly the direction to go and offers the reasons to choose one path, rather than another. Thus one may become more adept in avoiding routes that lead to frustrating dead ends.

In communication, nurses must fall back on their private resources—their emotions and intellect. Neither has to dominate the other; yet intellect may give the sturdiest support to the faltering. The more varied the theorectical resources, the sounder will be the resulting approaches.

Consider the disadvantages of seeing patients in only one perspective. Since no theory is of the "select-the-right-answer" school, there is an even chance that the nurse's knowledge will not pertain to the phenomena that it seeks to explain. Moreover, repetition of a single method that fails to achieve the desired results may lead to a sense of futility and bias against the patient. More problems, rather than insightful communication for problem solving, are likely to result when a patient's behavior is interpreted only in terms of its effects on the nurse. The resultant discord inevitably causes a breakdown in the communication process. Although the law of averages suggests that the nurse who has limited views of individuals must experience some degree of success from time to time and circumstances may be such that a given patient could tolerate such a frame of reference apparently without harm, dedication to one theory generally decreases the possibility of the nurse's providing the kind of help and support that is needed. From this brief digression the necessity for a multiple theoretical approach to understanding behavior may become more apparent.

When one is theorizing concerning the individual patient, the guidelines must be considered as probability statements only. A little reverence is in order so that we neither explain away what was communicated nor oversimplify the message. The patient's mental data-processing apparatus is subjective and thus beyond facile ideologic analysis. The concept of human diversity and dignity would have no meaning if only objective generalizations defined one's being. With this in mind the guidelines must always be flexible enough to accommodate new information, never obscuring the fact that separate pieces of patient behavior are still personal expressions of wholeness. From this insight the nurse may plan more meaningful intervention in helping the patient preserve his sense of intactness: structural, spiritual, and personal relatedness to his sociocultural environment. Although we are unable to "solve" the "puzzle" of each individual and pieces of behavior may be misleading and misunderstood, the available knowledge of human behavior may help us to unify the fragments better.

FIVE PERSPECTIVES OF HUMAN NATURE

There are many schools of thought concerning why people behave as they do.[1] Each theory has its ardent proponents, as well as opponents. Each differs in its basic assumptions, methods of observation, and conclusions. Concerning human affairs, each is imperfect in respect to its domain and to its declarations. Whatever the theoretical mintage, it will not be common currency for every human being. People tend to manifest a multitude of personal characteristics that seem to encompass all that is known and possibly a great deal that is unknown. Although human nature can be surveyed from many angles, this chapter will focus on the following points of view: psychoanalytic theory (with its premise that basic human nature is evil); behavioristic theory (that basic human nature is neutral); role theory (that basic human nature is neutral); humanistic theory (that basic human nature is good); and finally parapsychologic theory (that basic human nature is uncertain).

Psychoanalytic theory: Basic human nature is evil

Sigmund Freud is the best-known proponent of the theory that man is destined to behave in ways that are predetermined by three levels

of psychic life: the conscious, which is immediately focused in awareness; the subconscious, which is available to awareness at will; and
the unconscious, which contains those residues of past experiences
beyond recall. These strata of mental activity furnish the framework
for the three subsystems of the personality: the *id, ego,* and *superego.*[2]
The id, present at birth and throughout life, is part of and derived from
the unconscious. The ego, the largely conscious and social self, emerges
from the id after about the first 6 months of life as a result of the infant's
interaction with the environment. The superego operates on the unconscious level in opposition to the id and on the conscious level as the
"voice of conscience." Chronologically, the conscience develops last; beginning about the age of 5 years, it is not fully evolved until approximately the age of 10.

Central importance is given to the id because it is considered as the
source of all psychic energy. Its undisciplined, primitive, and biologic
urges are dichotomized into two conflicting drives: the life instinct, of
a sexual nature, and the death instinct, of an aggressive nature. The
id operates in terms of the pleasure principle or release of tension without regard to social consequences. Because the id is not restricted by
a sense of right or wrong, the domination of the person by these animal-
istic and amoral impulses is postulated to lead to a base nature. Furthermore, denial of man's base nature, instead of enobling him is believed
to simply make his behavior incomprehensible. Far from being self-
directive, man is motivated toward goals by thoughts and feelings related to material stored in his unconscious. Visible acts are not always
as voluntary as they seem. Sometimes the energetic id frees itself from
the control of the other parts of the personality and breaks through to
fulfill its wishes in dreams and unguarded slips of the tongue.

The ego is the "I," "me," or "myself" that distinguishes the person
from other human beings. The ego is the executive part of the personality, governing in a rational and reasonable manner such cognitive
functions as thinking, organizing, acting, and evaluating. The ego seeks
compromise between the unbridled impulses of the id and the inhibitions
of the superego by delaying or permitting gratification in accordance
with physical and social reality.

The superego computerizes and stores all the taboos, prohibitions,
ideals, and moral values that the child learned from significant others
during the process of socialization. This portion of the personality dictates in uncompromising ways what "ought to" be done and tries to
compel the ego to restrain desires judged to be wrong or evil. Real or
imagined transgressions may "hurt" one's conscience. Guilt is the retribution. However, the conscience may temporarily be anesthetized by
such drugs as alcohol, and for a while the released id can turn a listless
individual into the "life of the party."

Consider the functions that the ego must perform. Juxtaposed between the id and the superego, it must integrate the compulsions of these two warring factions and minimize intrapsychic conflict. Through intellectual resources the conscious self also seeks to mediate between the id and the external world, so that one can function in society in approved ways.

Prey to conflict from within and without, the individual uses mental mechanisms to eliminate or reduce the resultant tension and anxiety.[3] The concept of anxiety and defense mechanisms is one of the basic contributions of psychoanalytic theory to nursing; defense mechanisms are constantly used to communicate something of one's internal and external being.

The psychoanalytic theory may be summarized as follows: Behavior is determined by innate impulses and unconscious wishes and motivations. Although some environmental factors, especially parent-child relationships, have a significant effect, the major motivating forces are *instinctual* drives. Human beings have both constructive and destructive tendencies. Even though the ego tends toward rationality, the counterforces in the psyche, when coupled with early life experiences, are more conducive to irrational or evil deportment. On the group level, violence and war seem to support the assumption that human nature is basically irrational, aggressive, and destructive. Underlying our native endowment may be unresolved conflict.

Behavioristic theory: Basic human nature is neutral

Behaviorism, like psychoanalytic theory, regards free choice as largely an illusion—conduct is determined by forces beyond the individual's control—but here the similarity between the two schools of thought ends. Behaviorists explain personality development in terms of conditioning rather than as a reflection of inner experiences. To restate, human behavior is shaped by social indoctrination. Man's actions are believed to be as much automatic responses to *learning* as they are to symbolic expressions of unknown thoughts, feelings, and drives. Thus behaviorists prefer to concentrate on alleviating "specific symptoms rather than aiming at reorganizing the entire personality."[4] Moreover, behaviorists hold that the scientific measurement of observable behavior is the most valid means of formulating principles of human behavior.

In this view of behavior as being simply an integrated system of habits, emphasis is on the study of habits, particularly the manner in which they are learned, operate, and disappear. Basic concepts of this methodology are that the use of positive reinforcers (those which the person perceives as rewarding) can establish and promote behavior deemed adequate or desirable and that the use of negative reinforcers (those which the person perceives as punishing) can reduce or eliminate inadequate or undesirable behavior. Behaviorists conclude that basic human nature is neither bad nor good, rational nor irrational. How one behaves is dependent on positive or negative feedback from significant others; one has the neutral potential for either good or evil.

To effect behavioral changes, only the undesirable behavior is dealt with, since maladaptive behavior is postulated to be a consequence of maladaptive learning. This concept incorporates the learning theory that, when an established behavior pattern is no longer reinforced, it tends to be extinguished. People are helped to reach clear-cut, concise goals through the withdrawal of reinforcements.

The attainment of mutually derived goals in the nursing process may necessitate a change in patient behavior. Learning itself is but a change in behavior. When a patient is presented with new data and new ways of doing, some of the deterrents to proper functioning may be removed. Successful attainment of goals may be enhanced when the nurse has a theoretical point of view on how change can best be accomplished. Desired functioning may be facilitated when the nurse knows which responses to extinguish and which to encourage.

Behavior modification definitely involves language behavior. The nurse's interest, attention, and direct expressions of approval communicate to the patient that his behavior is "appropriate." In contrast, such negative reinforcers as failure to make a response or withholding eye contact communicate disapproval.

For illustrative purposes, suppose that a patient recovering from a stroke is reluctant to use his affected arm in the performance of activities of daily living. A mutual goal could be set for "encouraging use of the affected arm." In the event that the patient used, or attempted to use, this arm, the immediate feedback would be favorable. Whatever the reward—whether a smile, social conversation, or a cold glass of juice —it must have value to the patient. The rationale is that suitably rewarded behavior tends to recur. Conversely, if the nurse had to perform the activity in question, the positive reinforcers would be withheld. This time the nurse might remain silent during the activity and promptly leave after its completion. The lack of focus on the patient's feelings is justified by the supposition that (1) the more one is able to function independently, the greater the movement toward health and (2) a positive self-concept is fostered through the maximization of all one's potentials.

Behaviorism has its critics, as do other theories. Opponents are of the opinion that insensitivity to the reasons for the behavior, attitudes, and viewpoints of the patient concerning use of his affected arm will simply cause the feeling component of the behavior to present itself in yet another symptom.

Role theory: Basic human nature is neutral

"It's a boy!" "It's a girl!" With either of these affirmations of being, individuals are presumed to fall heir to several prearranged roles in an ongoing social system. From that point, they exist and develop their personalities in relation to those of others. Sex, culture, nationality, position in the family, and age, although not acquired by choice, promptly enmesh these helpless specimens of humanity in an intricately woven process of acculturation. Sullivan[5] believes that the individual in attempting to become part of the society into which he was born forms a "self-system," or basic appraisal of himself entirely under the influence of significant others. Emphasis is placed on anxiety, instead of intrapsychic forces, as the driving force in personality formation. Children learn to reject behavior that is displeasing to others so that they themselves will not be rejected. Beginning at a child's birth, parents, relatives, peers, teachers, clergy, and a host of others communicate the expected "way of doing"—the etiquette of behavior. So well is this lesson learned that in time it gains credence not only as the acceptable way but also as the *only* way of doing. Smooth social relations require what is called role reciprocity. Individuals are expected to behave in a manner compatible with their position and those of other group members.

Social role theory views the infant as a biologic tabula rasa: a clean slate for learning with untutored instincts for survival, such as searching for food. Accordingly, the infant is neither good nor bad but rather has a neutral set of capacities. This theory implies that one becomes "human" through the values, goals, attitudes, and mode of life that are communicated in the process of growing up. If appropriate behavior is learned from the complexity of interpersonal relationships, human affairs will be directed toward collaborative goals that offer mutual satisfaction and security.

Focus is on the implication that all understanding of self originates from the surroundings, that is, one's self-concept is profoundly affected by the reflected appraisal of others. Moreover, one estimates self-worth in terms of the degree of acceptance, rejection, or indifference communicated. Such appraisals of worth are imparted silently or audibly, consciously or unconsciously, actively or passively, and casually or formally within the context of interpersonal relationships. Generally, good mental health depends on the correspondence of one's self-perception to the perception that others have in regard to role behavior.

There are many ramifications to the premise that one's concept of personal merit only mirrors another's perception. From this standpoint, if significant others evaluate the individual as being worthless, bad, and irrational, subsequent behavior may well fulfill the prophecy. Low regard of another's worth may result in a traumatized psyche. Predictably, to question one's worth is to expect some form of protesting behavior in an interpersonal relationship; there can be as much identity in being *disliked* as in being *liked.*

Childhood is said to be a time when emotional and learning experiences have the greatest potentials. This is also the time when behavior is the most spontaneous, varied, and malleable. The child, in learning to become a functioning member of society, is most vulnerable to the effects of praise or blame. Also the child makes less distinction between the environment and self than does the adult. Through the labeling of behavior as *naughty, naughty* and reinforcing the displeasure with *shame on you,* the child is led to internalize an image of "the bad me." In contrast, behavior that is acceptable and socially sanctioned becomes part of the self-image of "the good me." Thus, while learning appropriate role behaviors, the very young learn to define themselves in relation to conduct that is permissible or forbidden. To this end, self-esteem becomes a consequence more of what one does than what one is, an exacting price to pay for interacting with others.

Various defense mechanisms must come into play to protect the self-system from too many devaluating judgments. By the same token, the more help one receives from the environment in developing a positive self-image, the more inner resources one has for mastery in role performances.

Three roles. During the embryonic stage of development the human being evolved from three primary germ layers: an inner layer (endoderm); a middle layer (mesoderm); and an outer layer (ectoderm).[6] Three distinct modalities of role behaviors analogous to the three germ layers are conceptualized: *the public self* (outer layer); *the private self* (middle layer); and the *ideal self* (inner layer). These versions of self are ascribed to the socialization process. The roles serve the purpose of helping the individual cope with the pressures of societal demands. How well one copes depends to a large extent on the harmonious integration of these three diverse layers into a unified self-system.

Public self. To continue the analogy, the outer layer, or public self, is synonymous with the ego, that part of man's personality that is shared and that projects an "image" of him in another's mind.[7] This self can assume multiple social roles, student, homemaker, widow, musician, and sweetheart. Because this is the part that others come to know best, this is also the part that the individual comes to know best in response to the judgments of others. The continuity of behavior in the roles helps reinforce self-perception and in this manner the public self confers identity. An example would be the person who retires after thirty or more years in the business world. The resultant loss of identity must be replaced to some degree with other reasons for living. Successful role performance unfortunately is evaluated in terms of societal needs. One is regarded as useful and normal only so long as performance in an essential role does not attract too many adverse notices.

Private self. Approximate to the middle layer is the private self. Equated to the id, this layer thus represents the unexpurgated version of people. Herein are said to be contained many personal characteristics that would interfere with smooth functioning in our public roles. The role behavior motivated by this layer is potentially unsharable and not for "polite society"; so this layer is subordinated by virtue of necessity.

Role theorists view the middle layer as essentially value free—neither good nor evil. Moreover, if there indeed exist specific instincts *necessary* for survival, this layer should be considered as *neutral*. However, its dimensions tend to be rather finite. Pressure and frustration can relegate too many forbidden impulses to this region of the mind. Understandably either external or internal relief of tension and anxiety must come.

There are many ways to "let off steam." Some people "blow their tops" in violent communication. Others may erode inwardly with ulcers and colitis. Still, many individuals find acceptable outlets in competitive sports. "Murder the bum" and "kill the umpire" are but verbal safety valves.

It is important to view this much maligned and repudiated portion of individuals in a different light, for only then can one understand and reconcile certain behaviors that are at odds with one's other roles. Indeed, this is a prerequisite for wholesome adjustments that make new modes of functioning possible. Perhaps the time has come to stop exclaiming after losing our tempers, "We don't know what came over us!"

Ideal self. Finally, there is the inner layer, one's ideal self. This layer seems to correspond to the superego, an intrinsic tribunal of "self-satisfaction or abasement."[8] Having been told from early childhood what one should or should not be like, one develops a concept of what one "ought" to be like. *Ought* implies such qualities as honor, courage, excellence, goodness, and creativity. Accompanying these oughts is the feeling that one is obliged to live up to certain expectations. These preconceived ideas support the mental image of the self one wishes to become. As a result, actual conduct often suffers in comparison to the ideal. Some persons express amazement at incongruence between idealization and action, for example, when profanity erupts as the balm for a stubbed toe. Resultant feelings of guilt seek expiation in apologies.

High value is placed on the ideal self, and its maintenance and enhancement are of the utmost importance in interpersonal relationships. For the potentialities of the ideal self to become actualities the public and private selves must cohere in a mutually sustaining symbiosis. Neither dimension should hold the individual in a tight, censorial grip—at best an energy-consuming exercise in futility. Recognizing one's short-comings, instead of denying them, leads to a type of knowledge that translates into self-improvement. The ideal self is just that—an abstraction of perfection. The most that one can do is to achieve a real self that strives to approach its potential for humaneness.

Social role of sickness. At times during the life cycle one is permitted to forgo a specific role with its usual social responsibilities. Illness offers such an exemption. However, commensurate with this respite from day-to-day obligations is the task of learning and adjusting to the new "sick role." This role has a prescribed common pattern of conduct: the patient is *expected* to cooperate with health personnel in the treatment of his condition.[9] Health care is predicated on reciprocal role behavior, primarily health practitioner initiative and patient receptivity. The patient's former self-concept and sense of autonomy, threatened by illness, may be radically altered by this turn of events.

Hospitalization is an "experience in distancing."[10] It places the individual who is ill a world apart from those who are healthy—in a foreign setting with strange artifacts, strange attire, and strange terminology. The distancing effect is compounded by isolation of the patient from his family and friends. Role expectations, coupled with diminution in strength and stamina, mandate passive and dependent modes of behavior. Individuals must passively submit to the most intimate, intrusive, often painful scrutiny and probing. On request, specimens from various systems must be produced for analysis. Similarly, to facilitate examinations, patients are instructed to "relax" while seminude. Unable to remove themselves physically, they resort to the natural use of body language: closing eyes and turning heads in vain attempts to shut out the intruders. This lack of regard from others reduces self-regard.

Another lesson inherent in the sick role is conformity to the institutional scheduling of time. There is a time to go to bed, to wake up, to wash up, and to have the bed made. People also find that they must increase their capacity for delaying gratification. They must learn to wait: in addition to waiting for recovery and discharge, they must wait for meals, medications, treatments, physician's rounds, nursing rounds, and visitors. Waiting involves much solitude and little certainty. One cannot be decisive while relying on the decisions of others. One is more likely to feel helpless and insecure. A sequel to such feelings is a lowered self-esteem.

In the rites de passage from person to patient, much identity is lost. People are numbered and the numbers securely affixed to their wrists. Recognition of individuality may be telescoped into "the liver problem, Bed 2, Room A-1118, Medical." Although these data may be sufficient to describe a patient, the *person* to whom it refers remains unknowable.

Despite the fact that this newly assigned identity is not meant to demean, it is an offense to one's sense of dignity.

Another vital and often overlooked aspect of the sick role is that one's sexuality is denied. The patient becomes a "nonperson" or sexual neuter. The nonperson is expected to have no reaction to intimate physical contact with nurses of the opposite sex. Such behavior, which in a social context would ordinarily bring censure, must be accepted matter-of-factly; but in any intimate interaction each participant is most decidedly aware of the other. Becoming inured to the presence of another is fairly impossible. Instead of reacting impersonally, one is more likely to be embarrassed, awkward, and anxious. One's feelings of worth diminish.

Another consequence of the sick role is lack of privacy. Privacy is usually reserved for the individual who is either affluent or terminally ill or who has a contagious disease. Privacy is not only an expensive commodity but also often in short supply. Generally, as far as privacy is concerned, rights are forfeited or waived. One must accommodate to the spatial privacy that is delimited by curtains or screens. Communication may be adversely affected; behavior becomes less spontaneous and more selective. Under such circumstances the patient takes care that only certain aspects of his being are made known. Since there is more need to keep up a facade, respect for the true self may decline.

Inherent in the sick role are many factors that do violence to one's self-concept. The anxiety that results is more likely to lead to regression than growth. Typically, the outcome of a lowered self-esteem is the tendency to seek solace in the middle layer, or private dimension, of one's being. When human beings are perceived in terms of symptoms and numbers, they have no choice but to relate in a manner that they think will be understood. To reassert identity, some become hostile, belligerent, and demanding.

Giving up their conventional ways of behavior, people tend to become more inner directed, concerned with symptoms and bodily functions. In the middle layer, instinctual behavior is dominant. Id behavior is directed toward keeping one's substance from becoming a silhouette. Inevitably, such self-absorption leads to antisocial behavior.

Unfortunately, the longer the sick role lasts, the greater the possibility for personality changes.[11] The person is no longer *the* liver problem but *a* liver problem. The number of visitors and frequency of visits tend to decline; roommates come and go; ward personnel change; the disease entity is no longer of special interest; and one may be in need of extensive care. Such patients may either be engaged in a struggle to maintain a sense of self or surrender what they are in a sense of futility.

Throughout life, there is always a delicate interplay between the psyche and the surroundings. Thus the self-concept is impervious to

neither time or space. It can become bruised and battered as it encounters the environment. Nurses should try to keep injuries to personal
integrity as low as possible. A good preventive measure is to provide
and maintain maximum interpersonal security for those who must occupy the sick role.

All roles are said to fill some societal function. Realistically this may
be the only way that highly structured institutions can run; yet what
is ingenious is not necessarily just. No role should require human beings
to become passive automatons. Patients should not have to become non-
persons by default. A viable alternative is redefining the sick role so
that it is made more personal in personally acceptable ways, with individuals' needs dictating role behavior as much as possible. To accomplish this is to modify the existing "oughts" of sick role behavior, so
that people do not become caricatures of themselves.

Humanistic theory: Basic human nature is good

Humanism promotes a positive regard for people.[1] Thus it differs
with the behavioristic, the psychoanalytic, and in some measure the
role theory of behavior. To begin with, behaviorists need to balance their
concern for observable behavior with some concern for individuals.
Presently these theories carefully avoid the particulars of the emotions.
To pursue the matter further, psychoanalytic models of behavior present
too uncompromising appraisals of human beings. So far as behavior
is concerned, at birth the "die is cast" in the direction of negativism
and irrationality. Role theory places excessive emphasis on regimen-
tation of human life. When people are imprisoned in rigid scenarios,
they may well become reactive puppets, instead of active participants
in shaping their own destinies. What is needed is more social generosity.
The environment should nourish one's uniqueness and set the stage for
choices of behavior.

Humanism emphasizes the person's capabilities within a broad range
of possibilities. In other words, a person is capable of a variety of actions
that are polarized: good or evil and rational or irrational, depending on
the ways in which their abilities are encouraged or frustrated. Humanists explain that man's natural propensity is to "unify his energy" in
the search for meaning and a sense of purpose in life and to "walk
as far as he can to its frontiers."[12] In a supportive setting, human affairs
operate nearer the poles of goodness and rationality. Even with handicaps and deprivation, individuals often rise above adversity in a com-
mendable fashion. Basically, then, the innermost core—the "id," or private self—contains laudable, humane qualities for purposive human
strivings.

These controversial aspects of basic human nature have significant impact on interpersonal relationships. If people are innately masochistic and predatory, what must follow is stringent control for "one's own good" and "the good of society." No allowances are made for self-direction and self-fulfillment. On the other hand, if one adopts a neutral or positive view of human nature, societal values should not be blindly accepted. Rather society should foster those tendencies, which humanists hold as given, that lead to responsible self-determination and self-actualization.

Maslow's model of basic human needs. Maslow has incorporated the goal-directed behavior toward self-actualization into a sequential arrangement of need priorities.[13] One's self-concept influences the potency of each need, as well as the goals set for fulfillment. Since the self-concept is dynamically involved, the degree to which needs are appropriately gratified depends in some measure on interpersonal relationships.

One can recognize a sequential ordering of needs, from the lowest ones of self-defense to the highest one of self-enhancement. The hierarchy can be helpful if seen as an interrelated system of communicating "physiological needs, safety needs, needs for love and belonging, esteem needs, and the need for self-actualization."[14] This is more apparent when one considers that an acute, unmet need leads to energetic action, as the person seeks ways to satisfy the need or to decrease its strength. Commanding most of the individual's attention, unmet needs are communicated to us in a diversity of behaviors.

Often the individual may be unaware or only partially aware of what the needs are. Unless further clarification is given, the need may never be known. By keeping in mind the five basic human needs, one may better identify what the individual is lacking.

Basic human needs are positioned in ascending order comparable to normal growth and development. Once a lower need is met, one on the next higher level is said to take its place. The higher the need, the greater the demand for social maturity. However, on any level the thwarting of a need that the person considers a priority can lead to inner frustration and outer conflict.

The *physiologic needs* are self-preservation and reproduction. They maintain life and perpetuate the species. Thus if one requires food, water, and sleep, any nursing activity unrelated to reasonably satisfying these needs is likely to be irrelevant.

Second to the physiologic needs is the psychologic *need for security*. This can be described as the desire to feel safe in a stable environment that affords protection from physical and psychic harm. A dependable and trustworthy setting has order, instead of chaos; predictability, instead of uncertainty; and familiarity, instead of strangeness.

When the physical and psychologic needs are fairly well satisified, the *need for love and belonging* emerges. Each person needs to attain interpersonal companionship in either family or friendship groups. Loving, close ties with others are especially important in times of crisis and may also help to diminish the effects of socioeconomic hardships that might pose impregnable barriers to self-actualization.

The fourth need is for achievement, maintenance, and enhancement of *self-esteem.* It is the desire to be able to give a "good account" of oneself. A positive identity is exemplified by feelings of worth, adequacy, compentency, and usefulness. The higher the self-evaluation, the less dependent one is one the appraisal of others. The higher one's regard for self, the more strength and confidence one has to cope with the vicissitudes of life.

The last need in the hierarchy is *self-actualization.* This concept is more difficult to assess. It describes *ongoing* tendencies that do not fit easily into other theories of behavior. This need differs from the other four in that it is not involved in maintaining biologic, psychologic, or social equilibrium. In fact, the independent initiative that is characteristic of the satisfaction of this need can lead to risky ventures, such as climbing Mt. Everest and crossing the Atlantic in a sailboat. Self-actualizing people seem to have come to terms with themselves and face life as unified wholes. Since less energy is spent in meeting lower needs, they can make optimum use of their capacities and resources for creative self-expression of values that give true meaning to existence.

Humanists believe that the universal upward-striving qualities in people are often underrated. Such underestimation of individuals deprives them of their natural rights for growth, autonomy, and self-realization and in effect often denies them the use of their resources, capacities, and talents for reaching goals. In her desire to be helpful the nurse may "overdo" and block the emergence of these striving qualities. This may explain why some patients seem ungrateful no matter what is done for them. *The reality may be that the nurse is meeting her own needs, rather than the patient's.* From this viewpoint, helping patients to help themselves while striving toward health takes into account human life's highest aspirations, that is, the innate need for growth and maximal use of potentials. Self-actualization does not mean freedom from discomfort. There is often pain; but, in view of the alternatives, this approach to patient care is in the end the most humane.

Complete gratification of a lower need does not guarantee movement to a higher level of functioning. Need satisfaction could well have, as a consequence, inertia, disinterest, and ennui; yet behavior that leads to mature growth is based on the fact that human beings are always "wanting." In this light, most of us may function best when something is deficient. However, some needs, such as safety, esteem, and belonging, have become nursing values, and patients likely require some assistance in meeting their physiologic needs. However, in reality often the most important goal is sustaining the personal resources and incentives of individuals, so that they can gratify their needs according to their own value system.

Parapsychology: Basic human nature is uncertain

How can we speak of uniqueness without recognizing the assumption that individuals are capable of cognitive behaviors that go beyond the explanations of well-known and deeply entrenched theories? How incoincidental must something be before it is seen as other than a coincidence? These are some of the issues that parapsychologists are seeking to resolve. Serious efforts are being made to fit a variety of unusual human activities under some type of plausible theoretical umbrella. Beneath this is a potpourri of extraordinary experiences that the usual psychologic and physical factors do not explain. Such behaviors range from telepathy, precognition, mental healing, out-of-body experiences, and seeing auras and apparitions to communicating with spirits, just to mention a few.

Unfortunately, much of the current research has depended on human testimony that cannot withstand human critique. These improbable events or reputed abilities compel a lot of interest, as well as disbelief. Man's deeper needs for primitive magic pose great difficulty in separating fact from fancy; these extraordinary experiences are unusually resistant to voluntary repetition or laboratory replication. Thus parapsychologists are accused of taking more liberties than is scientifically permissible, since the derived theories are based more on speculation than experimentation.

Still, although parapsychology is viewed with skepticism, any system of thought suggesting that we have not reached the limits of knowledge concerning human behavior should not summarily be dismissed. Skepticism does not reject the new in the name of objectivity and may be the scholar's most useful approach in the application of any methodology. Most theories concerning man may be at best only provisionally useful and ever subject to revision. We must remember that our primary commitment is to existence, rather than to the theories purporting to explain it.

It is axiomatic that the brain has vast resources of which we are unaware. People have unused and unimagined potential. This latent power has been hypothesized as existing in yet *another self*—"the subliminal self," which "represents more fully our central and abiding being."[15] This self is further subdivided into regions analogous to the unconscious but is said to be of such scope that it can never find complete expression through normal corporeal manifestations. Because some part of the subliminal self is always unmanifested, man has mental powers held in abeyance or reserve. Sometimes the heterogeneous mix of supernormal cognition from one of the segments of this psychic spectrum emerges through organs partly trained for their performance: hands for automatic writing, eyes for visions and apparitions, ears for hallucinatory voices, speech for mediumistic-trances, and thoughts for thought transference.

Paranormal phenomena may contain a complex "reality" that was formerly felt to be peculiar to the mentally disturbed. Perception is ever subject to the internal vigilance of the ego. All perceptions cannot be consciously acknowledged. Many images that emanate from the environment must be excluded from awareness or given "selective inattention." Otherwise, constant distraction by trivial details would interfere with one's attending to those aspects of the surroundings that are significant for one's purpose. Effective though our sense organs may be as filters of extraneous stimuli, conscious unawareness does not mean that what was unnoticed went unregistered; and there is no guarantee that what was perceived will be faithfully reproduced. Familiar information may be organized into new relationships—into a new way of knowing, or extrasensory perception. Naturally the rational self seeks to erect defense, against the anxiety that develops whenever the ego is endangered by forces inconsistent with the familiar scheme of things. For comfort as well as convenience we simply interpret these phenomena as intuition.

However, some forces can overcome the normal ego defenses and bypass the recognized channels of communication. When the usual mode of entry is effectively blocked, a telepathic process, or "thought transference" may occur, particularly if the relationship or the message is emotionally charged.[16] As an instance most of us can "sense" when we are being stared at. Mind-to-mind communication has been defined as the process wherein the "brain of one person can impose its rhythms on the brain of another" and influence the other's state of mind and physical processes.[17] Surely this is sufficient reason to reject the notion of mental telepathy. Hearing what others have to say is bad enough; be thankful that we have some protection from their thoughts.

We do not, however. The unknowing individual may be bombarded with a host of telepathic impressions from those close by that could conceivably cause fluctuations in mood, temperament, and health status.[18] The mind may not easily repel alien thoughts, as the body repels foreign tissue. The lay public seems adept in reducing pretentious formulations to perceptive aphorisms; a fairly probable conclusion is that a person can be affected by "good or bad vibrations" from another. More consideration might be given to the possibility that positive attitudes toward patients may help to create therapeutic climates. Deep feelings of goodwill are postulated to become self-transcending. The self-transcendent nature of the event can cause a transition of emotions from the conscious to the subliminal level, at which the message may find a route for mind-to-mind expression. Who among us has not been thinking of a song only to hear another hum it? and what accounts for two persons' speaking the same phrases at the same time?

Healing, whether by divinity, doctors, or voodoo, is a process that is incompletely understood. A patient's will and faith have long been accepted to be positive contributors. Since this is agreed, perhaps the time has come for science and superstition to become better acquainted. Any ability possessed by man may be improved with practice; the task of body repair is no exception. Deep concern for a patient can circumvent the normal paths of verbal and nonverbal communication and cause him to rally by increasing his "resistance to pathology" and generally "strengthening his immunological system."[19] Evidence suggests that there is "some energy flow" from healer to patient and that this transmission may take place when the healer is not in the patient's presence.[19] It may take place in relationships of goodwill when one is completely unaware. One could also speculate that telepathy helps account for the differences in response that a patient has to essentially the same nursing care.

Of all the paranormal phenomena, precognition seems to make us the most uncomfortable. Precognition challenges our very notion of time —that which is measurable in days, hours, minutes, and seconds. Events are routinely ordered sequentially into a undirectional dimension of past, present, and future. Pause for a moment to consider the concept called the *present.* So certain are we that we know what it means that any definition other than *now* seems superfluous, as may also be the question, "What are you doing now?" If you reply, "I am reading," a perplexing situation arises: for the instant that the printed symbol evokes a mental image, you have *read.* You may continue reading, but each time that a word is perceived by the brain, what you say you *are* currently doing has already been *done.* Thus the present and our concept of time is neither scientific nor very sophisticated. Moreover, if the present exists at all, how can one define it other than by saying that it is partly one's past and partly one's future. Man's subliminal self is said to have much knowledge about the future, and this awareness breaks through when he is off guard. Sometimes it takes the form of a vivid dream, a graphic vision, or a sudden flash. Often the individual experiences vague feelings of uneasiness, along with the certain knowledge of impending doom.

More than chance occurrence is the case of the patient who calmly announces his death before any signs are apparent. Such patients seem to be in a state of spiritual-emotional detachment from life and do not fit the customary dying trajectory, or the expected course of dying for persons with similar conditions. With the desire neither to fight nor flee, the patient's prediction often comes true within 24 hours.[20] Because the patient's information is so difficult to assimilate, we may be tempted disdainfully to make light of his "knowing." The patient, himself, seems unable to offer any clarification other than that he "just knows!" Our need for rationality and order makes this kind of communications particularly disturbing. We like to know why; certified causes of death make it more comprehensible. Sudden death reminds us too much of our own precarious mortality, especially if the signs cannot be medically monitored. Although we bandy about such terms as *scared to death,* there is a deep human disbelief that powerful emotions can contribute to or directly cause death. Just as the individual who is completely determined to commit suicide cannot be stopped, perhaps the patient convinced that he is going to die cannot be saved; but we do not know. We do know that our current system of helping resources seems inadequate. We should let our ignorance detain us at least long enough to learn from such patients. When we cling to the familiar, we cease to advance toward new horizons of helping. These patients must not be left to face so many imponderables alone. Parapsychology reminds us more than do other theories that uniqueness also means to be remarkably one of a kind.

Theories as sources of understanding

To recapitulate, understanding human behavior is one of the basic requirements of effective communication. However, this understanding itself is not sufficient. Communication in nursing is the synthesis of artistry and knowledge. One's signature is put to both only when the two skills are put to use. Consequently, the final yardstick of understanding must be its application.

An understanding of human behavior channels observations so that relationships that may not be readily apparent to others are seen. To illustrate, patients tend to complain of more pain at night than during the day. Nurses who are not on their theoretical toes may interpret this behavior as a need for medication. Various other aspects of causation may not be weighed. In contrast, knowledge of human behavior helps the nurse to account for this behavior from different points of view. She would be less inclined to resolve the problem by putting the patient to sleep. This "cure" has the same life span as does the insomnia. Patients may or may not need medication. Certainly other possibilities should be explored.

First, the nurse could observe for physical manifestations of the patient's emotional state. Perhaps a message other than pain is being communicated through body language. If the patient is huddled in bed facing the wall, head bowed, shoulders sagging, maybe there is an overwhelming burden that he needs to share. Pain may be a plea for help—for something other than a pill. The nurse needs to understand the covert meaning of pain complaints. Consider the impact of sensory deprivation on human behavior. Diminished sensory input may make the nights long, lonely hours of social isolation; visitors, telephones, radios, reading, and television may be forbidden. When stimulation by the usual sounds, visual perceptions, and tactile sensations is drastically curtailed, the patient may experience disabilities unrelated to his organic condition.[21] Impairment of intellectual processes, perceptual distortions such as hallucinations, and gross disturbances in feeling states are not uncommon consequences of prolonged absence of adequate stimuli. Aloneness may cause persons to focus inward; decreased sensory input increases self-perception. Not surprisingly, the perception of pain may be heightened. The nurse may wish to increase the sensory input via sight, sound, or touch. Manipulation of external conditions may distract the patient, so that the pain can be better tolerated or temporarily go unnoticed.

The nurse also needs to direct attention toward sociocultural factors. Response to pain is presumed to be a learned behavior that varies according to age, sex, cultural group, and past experience.[22] Society has conditioned the male to be less emotionally expressive regarding pain than is the female. The nurse also needs to understand that illness may cause regression to a previous level of behavior that brought satisfaction. Complaints of pain can have secondary gain—attention—by bringing the nurse and sometimes the physician to the bedside. The patient now has companionship, and the need that motivated the behavior becomes less intense. Pain, like many complaints, can symbolically communicate what cannot be voiced. Successful treatment cannot ignore the communicative aspects of pain.

Further narrowing down the pain complaint, the nurse knows that pain reminds individuals of their mortality as nothing else can. What follows is that the most significant emotion attached to pain is anxiety. Pain is but rarely perceived as good; more often it is viewed as a warning of something dreadful. Night accentuates this dread; people know that more deaths occur at night than during the day. Realizing that security is one of the basic human needs, the nurse may place priority on the relief of anxiety, rather than the relief of a physical symptom. Moreover, decreasing one's anxiety increases one's tolerance for pain. Medication, if needed, may be given in a smaller dose and be more effective.

Notice also that gastric secretions tend to peak at night. In conditions such as peptic ulcers, pain starts when the stomach is empty.[23] This finding would be most significant in terms of diagnosis and treatment. In this case the nursing action would be to *defer* giving medication that would mask significant symptoms.

Yet another approach is available to the nurse who desires to help a patient sleep comfortably at night. Thought could be given to decreasing the "buzzer-pushing actions" through behavioral modification. However, in this instance the nurse's behavior might well be the factor that is modified.

Time now for reflection: the nurse can look back to see what happened, look at what is currently happening, or look forward to see what can be done next. Here the "placebo effect" may well be considered. An inactive substance given in the form of an injection or pill (placebo) is known to be able to alleviate pain. Placebo responders are often thought to be malingerers and not as sick as the person who requires potent analgesics. This is not so.

Faith in the nurse and what she is trying to do to help may be sufficient stimulus to mobilize the spirit in a patient, organizing his body and personality more efficiently against disintegration.[24] Relief of pain, if strongly and sincerely wished for, can be accomplished not only by pharmacologic means but "rather through the impact of man-on-man mediated through the patient's perceptual-cognitive structure."[24] This kind of telepathic input may also augment the other approaches and sustain the patient until one or more of the other therapies work.

Understanding human behavior can help the nurse to make tentative predictions about groups of patients. In fact, sensory deprivation at night has many parallels during the day. To illustrate, many patients, because of the nature of their conditions, are placed in isolation. Too often they are left bereft of the companionship of other human beings if one excludes the occasional forays by nurses. The room itself is likely to be away from "ward traffic." Isolation can be an existence steeped in monotony. Thus one should anticipate that whatever physical or emotional discomforts patients have will be magnified. There is also a need for increased awareness of the effects of sensory deprivation in everyday life. The boredom of monotonous tasks and turnpike driving may accelerate the rate of accidents.

To conclude, theories in and of themselves are only visions of understanding, and their acuity can be validated only in practice.

REFERENCES

1. Thompson, C.: The different schools of psychoanalysis, American Journal of Nursing **57**:1304-1307, 1957.
2. Freud, S.: New introductory lectures on psychoanalysis, (Strachey, E., editor), New York, 1965, W. W. Norton & Co., Inc., p. 72.
3. Mereness, D., and Taylor, C.: Essen-

tials of psychiatric nursing, St. Louis, 1974, The C. V. Mosby Co., pp. 46-51.

4. Cadoret, R., and King, L.: Psychiatry in primary care, St. Louis, 1974, The C. V. Mosby Co., p. 249.

5. Sullivan, H.: The psychiatric interview, New York, 1954, W. W. Norton & Co., Inc., p. 101.

6. Langman, J.: Medical embryology, Baltimore, 1963, The Williams & Wilkins Co., p. 29.

7. James, W.: Psychology: a briefer course, New York, 1961, Harper & Row, Publishers, p. 46.

8. *Ibid.,* p. 57.

9. Vincent, P.: The sick role in patient care, American Journal of Nursing **75:**1172-1173, 1975.

10. Montesinos, J.: Spanish for nurses, New York, 1976, Borough of Manhattan Community College Press, p. 2.

11. Sorenson, K., and Amiss, D.: Understanding the world of the chronically ill, American Journal of Nursing **67:**811-817, 1967.

12. Fromm, E.: The anatomy of human destructiveness, New York, 1973, Holt, Rinehard & Winston, Inc., p. 267.

13. Maslow, A.: Toward a psychology of being, New York, 1968, Van Nostrand Reinhold Co., p. 199.

14. Ibid., pp. 199-200.

15. James, W.: What psychical research has accomplished. In Van Over, R., editor: Psychology and extrasensory perception, New York, 1972, The New American Library, Inc., p. 84.

16. Eisenbud, J.: The use of the telepathy hypothesis in psychotherapy. In Bychowski, G., and Despert, J., editors: Specialized techniques in psychotherapy, New York, 1952, Grove Press, Inc., p. 46.

17. Ostrander, S., and Schroeder, L.: Psychic discoveries behind the iron curtain, Englewood Cliffs, N.J., 1970, Prentice-Hall, Inc., p. 231.

18. Panati, C.: Supersense: our potential for parasensory experience, New York, 1974, The New York Book Co., p. 111.

19. Ibid., p. 82.

20. Walker, M.: The last hour before death, American Journal of Nursing **73:**1592-1593, 1973.

21. Hebb, D.: The mammal and his environment, Journal of Psychiatry **111:**826, 1955.

22. Macaffrey, M., and Moss, F.: Nursing intervention for bodily pain, American Journal of Nursing **67:**1224-1227, 1967.

23. Lon, B.: Sleep, American Journal of Nursing **69:**1896-1899, 1969.

24. Jourard, S.: The transparent self, New York, 1964, D. Van Nostrand Co., p. 89.

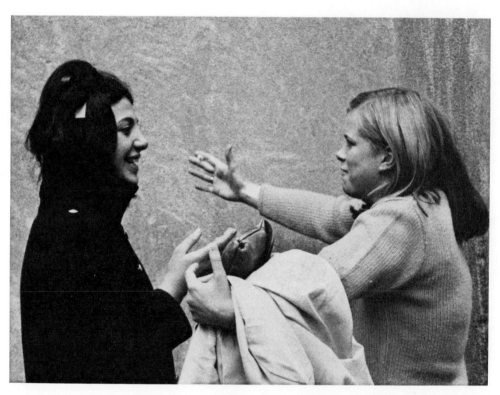

Characteristic of human beings is purposeful, *goal-directed*, behavior. Many human activities of deep personal meaning may not involve dialogue. Feelings, attitudes, and emotions may be conveyed through the medium of body language. Effective interactions are contingent on mastery and synchronization of the many shadings and subtleties of cues and clues in the syntax of *silent language*. (Photograph by Berne Greene, Editorial Photocolor Archives.)

CHAPTER 3

Keys to understanding and being understood

OVERVIEW

In human interactions, man's greatest achievement is his audible and silent language. Within the constraints of words and gestures he thinks, feels, judges, and acts. A large part of a person's behavior seems to be concerned with transmitting and receiving messages. Talking, listening, thinking, reading, and writing can occupy many of his waking hours. In sleep, man's private self communicates by tossing and turning; grinding his teeth; talking; and, in rare instances, sleepwalking. Communication and living are inextricable; man's survival in a fluctuating world has been said to depend on his "capacity to collect, process and use information."[1]

When one contrasts the technologic advancements in communication with the slender progress toward truly effective interpersonal communication, the cultural lag is awesome. Computers can collect, process, transmit, and store prodigious amounts of data with incredible precision and speed. For this reason, computers have emerged as a major influence in our lives and are used to communicate with large numbers of people. With computer-based information centers the attempt has been made to reduce men's personhood to microfilm, but what he truly was, is, or can be cannot thus be postulated. With electronic tools we categorize, mechanize, and quantify life without the value of humaneness, ignoring the fact that the most important aspects of existence are in the human area. The cultural lag exists because technology, the omnipresent maker of tools, has not yet become the omnipotent shaper of man. Thus interpersonal communication must resist rather than follow the technologic orientation toward people, since "no equation can divine the quality of life, no instrument record, no computer conceive it . . . only bit by bit can feeling man lovingly retrieve it."[2] The special quality of life is human dignity; through interpersonal communication, dignity is given meaning.

Interpersonal communication is a shared process of transmitting "facts, feelings and meanings by words, gestures, or other actions."[3] The process is circular. In a simplified way this circuit may be described in terms of four elements: the sender, the message, the receiver, and feedback to the sender. The four elements are, however, versatile and vexatious media for the challenging and complex interplay of one human mind with another. Success of communication in the patient-nurse relationship depends on the nurse's knowing what she is trying to convey, the purpose of her message, communicating what she really means to the patient, and comprehending the meaning of what the patient is intentionally or unintentionally communicating to her. The success of such an interdependent activity may be evaluated in terms of the degree to which each participant understands what was communicated and can "communicate this understanding to the other's satisfaction" verbally or nonverbally.[4]

PATIENTS' NEEDS AND THERAPEUTIC COMMUNICATION

Professionals in a calling based on helping must change with the changing needs of those whom they seek to help. In nursing the most common and urgent needs of patients seem to be increasingly emotional in nature, although the majority of patient-nurse relationships are a direct consequence of illness. Research has shown that the hospitalized patient's communication has two primary objectives: securing information and interpersonal contact.[5] Unless the patient received the desired information concerning his illness and the procedures and social organization of the hospital, his anxiety level tended to be high. He also evidenced needs for someone to talk to, to keep him from feeling isolated and lonely, to be kind to him, and to give emotional support. Critically significant to the nursing process is the belief that the more that is known and shared about the patient—his physical, psychologic, spiritual, and sociocultural functioning—the more effective will be his therapeutic regimen.[6] A renowned sociologist observed that members of a profession "tend to invest their egos primarily in certain routines, giving less stress to the other ones which they perform."[7] When interacting with "clients," the professional infuses activities with signs that dramatically highlight competence not in a variety of routines "but only with the one from which his occupational reputation derives."[7] The corollary to the nursing profession, Whiting[8] concluded from his study is that of all the nursing activities of relative importance, those ranked highest by nurses concerned medications.

Nurses, according to another observer, are proficient in carrying out specific, detailed, and routinized actions to alleviate physical discomfort but deficient in dealing with the emotional aspects of illness in such a manner that the results of their intervention will be more effective and long lasting.[9] The problems that nurses experience with patients seem to relate not so much to giving task-oriented physical care as to communication, or a lack of awareness that patients have problems in other areas that are as vital to recovery as are the more traditionally defined medical procedures. Thus, in meeting the needs of patients, the nurse seems primarily to need unprecedented levels of excellence in communication.

Therapeutic regimens and communication must consolidate. In Ruesch's opinion a prerequisite to therapeutic communication is "the presence of another person who understands, acknowledges, and responds to the patient."[10] Such characteristics in the nurse are essential to purposeful professional conversation that enables the nurse to know her patients as special human beings with individual needs. Whenever the nurse converses with the patient to obtain information so that her intervention will be personalized and maximally helpful, she is communicating with the patient therapeutically.[11]

Therapeutic communication may be thought of as interviewing, "since any goal-directed contact with patients constitutes an interview."[12] However, unlike an interview in the strict sense of the word, therapeutic communication may take place *informally* in conjunction with other nursing activities as well as *formally* in taking a nursing history of patients when they are admitted to the health care setting.

KEYS: WHAT THEY ARE AND WHAT THEY CAN DO

If therapeutic communication is to accomplish its objectives, one needs an overall strategy to guide endeavors. Keys are interviewing strategies, principles, or techniques that facilitate understanding of oneself and others. Keys aid in unlocking doors that obscure the patient's immediate needs. Keys aid in helping him to communicate his needs and in helping the nurse to meet those needs. Unless the nurse knows the patient's needs, she cannot help him, and she cannot know his needs unless the patient discloses them to her. Keys are general, rather than standardized, methods of professional communication. They are "skeletal" in the sense that they are "fleshed out" by the nurse's practice. The nurse may find that some keys are suitable and that others suit neither her nor the situation; hence there is no "master key" or infallible technique.

When the nurse first practices interviewing techniques, she may feel uneasy and self-conscious. Continued and diligent practice is one means of gaining proficiency and self-confidence. Fearing that the use of principles may detract from the art of communication, some nurses may bridle at the very mention of "professional conversation." Although warmth, concern, friendliness, and spontaneity are essential to the art of communication, they are also compatible with knowledge. The warm, concerned, friendly, and spontaneous nurse needs also to be well informed.

Concern and knowledge must function in concert. The demanding patient affords an excellent example. To want to help a patient whose behavior indicates that he desperately needs help and not know how can be a frustrating, even devastating experience for the nurse, who becomes frustrated and angry "not because the demanding patient makes her work harder, but because the nurse never feels successful in meeting his needs."[12] As a result the nurse may avoid the patient, and communication breaks down. Conversely, the knowledgeable nurse may be warm and friendly as a result of her knowledge that an individual's behavior may be caused by unconscious forces over which he has no control. She demonstrates concern by remaining with the patient even though the situation may be difficult and unpleasant. She uses interviewing techniques that may assist in discovering the patient's needs at the moment. The nurse uses her true self therapeutically with the realization that to help is to communicate interest and compassion— to stand by and to listen. The art and science of communication make up human caring, which may be all that the patient needs at the moment.

The nurse's spontaneity need not be suppressed by rigid interpersonal behavior. Still, spontaneity is inhibited by respect. Impulsively saying and doing the first thing that comes to mind is one means of erecting barriers to communication. The nurse must be cautious not to misjudge the importance of the patient's problem either by making light of a serious problem or by magnifying what may be a minor one. If the patient thinks that the nurse has showed disregard for his feelings, he will be unlikely to disclose himself further. Yet spontaneity may be a valuable humanistic asset when combined with a faculty for appropriateness. Once a sense of what is fitting is internalized, the nurse's natural style of self-expression may be as effective as it is distinctive.

WHEN STRANGERS MEET

Sometimes a nurse may obtain much relevant information about a given patient from her colleagues. Still, such information is not the final word about a patient's personality, and the nurse's initial encounter with the patient is essentially stranger-to-stranger, for she needs to validate what she has previous learned accurately by her own observations of the patient as he is now. When strangers meet, whether or not they have some prior knowledge of each other, they interact according to their unique frames of reference or the personal standards and values that underlie their attitudes and actions. Both are egocentric. During the process of getting acquainted, specific concepts about the individual often derive from one's assumptions about people in general. Zunin and Zunin concluded from their observations that during the "hello" phase of a relationship in our culture there is an average time of "four minutes" in which one must overcome the "initial turbulence of the psyche in the human frame of reference."[13] The concepts that each person forms of the other determine the degree to which strangers make contact and collaborate toward goals. In long-term patient-nurse relationships what happens in the first few minutes is not irreversible, but, when the relationship is a short-term one, the positive potential to create "response and involvement, to give and take, talk and listen, to communicate," may be jeopardized or lost.[14]

A prerequisite to understanding is an accurate "patient-concept," which Jourard defined as "the nurse's assumptions or beliefs about the patient."[15] This impression of the patient, whether right or wrong, finds expression in the nurse's behavior. Unless she acquires a concept of her patient that is accurate and up to date, from the beginning to the end of the patient-nurse relationship the nurse will likely have "been treating a person whom she does not know."[15]

Frequently, inaccurate concepts may be formed of another on the basis of "surface language," or observable characteristics. This first step in responding is akin to "reconnoitering," a kind of surveying with one's senses. Endless numbers of inferences are made on the basis of such characteristics as height, weight, complexion, hairstyle, age, diction, dress, body odor, tone of voice, and vocabulary. That people can form positive or negative concepts on the basis of observable traits was documented by Thornton in a study of the effects of wearing eyeglasses.[16] Participants in the study uniformly judged strangers wearing glasses to be more intelligent, industrious, and serious than those not wearing glasses.

When communicating with strangers, one needs to consider two contradictory concepts. A simple restatement of the first is that "birds of a feather flock together," and therefore likeness enhances communication. The second is that "opposites attract," in which case the needs of the participants would be complementary and communication also enhanced. Not surprisingly, Byrne's study supports the first concept, that the greater the number of identical factors, the greater the cohesion of interest and the less the discord in communication.[17] A stranger with like needs, attitudes, intellect, and observable characteristics was more positively regarded by the study group than was a stranger who was dissimilar in these areas. What was surprising, however, were the negative conjectures that the stranger who differed was less socially responsible, moral, and well adjusted.

In day-to-day transactions we do not as a matter of course conduct our affairs scientifically. We live by assumptions in functioning as members of groups, organizations, and society. An individual riding the same bus to work daily, as a passenger, has confidence that the bus driver will follow the same route. Not subjecting the event to statistical probabilities, the passenger has no way of determining if this will indeed be so and in fact does not know for a certainty that the bus driver will even allow him to board. However, the assumption is made that he will be a passenger and that the driver will follow the same route. The assumptions, in time, may be substituted for facts.

The nurse inevitably makes assumptions about the patient when the two first interact. As they become better acquainted, the initial patient concept provides valuable data that can be tested for accuracy and progressively revised by further observation. However, since first impressions are said to be untempered by time, it is vitally important that the nurse's earliest appraisal of the patient be as accurate as possible. If her original estimate of the "face value" of an individual proves to be correct, effective communication and joint social action is made possible. On the other hand, if the nurse misjudges a patient and makes no further inquiry into his individuality, the human enterprise is built on a set of false expectations with the patient bearing the burden of proving himself a worthy partner.

Although additions and modifications of the nurse's primary assumptions concerning the patient occur as the relationship develops, retaining the illusion of being "a pretty good judge of character" seems to be essential to ego functioning. Thus only those later developments which support, rather than contradict, primary opinions are likely to be acknowledged, for who among us is willing to reverse an opinion by admitting that his unique frame of reference is a refuge for false assumptions?

Because the patient may be unable to meet his needs unaided, his dependency may make him hesitate to risk open conflict with the nurse to alter the relationship once it is under way; and, if the interaction is to present at least a surface agreement, the patient's facade will be one of silence or noncommitment on matters of relevance to him. In essence he forfeits what he is and is thus responded to in terms of what he is assumed to be. If a patient does not have the freedom to interact with the nurse in ways that facilitate communication, even though the relationship projects a veneer of understanding, it will be one of estrangement.

Before an interpersonal relationship can truly commence, the nurse and patient must reach a common ground of receptivity to each other. A time factor in which social pleasantries may mask the true drama

of first encounters seems to be involved. Diverse communication techniques are needed in initiating a relationship, and continued diversity
and skills in communication are needed if the patient-nurse relationship
is to be positively ongoing because the patient's behavior changes as
his needs change. The lower physiologic and safety needs may be gratified with minimum communication, but, once these needs are met, a
higher need gains potency. These more subtly expressed needs of patients seem to require greater nursing expertise in communication. Of
all the needs, said Eric Fromm, man's greatest is the "need to overcome
his separateness, to leave the prison of his aloneness," to be loved—to
belong.[18]

THE SETTING

The conditions under which an interview takes place may significantly affect communication. Although Garrett states that the "physical
setting of the interview may determine its entire potentiality," in nursing the traditional office setting is a rarity.[19] More vital than the physical
layout, furnishing, and decor is orienting the individual to the surroundings, so that they become more predictable and safe. When a patient
enters the hospital, he is in unfamiliar territory. Because of the nurses'
24-hour presence the wards are considered to be their domain.[20] This
preeminence of nurses is reinforced by the less frequent appearance
of physicians and administrators. Perceiving himself as an unwelcome
interloper, the patient "becomes timid and apologetic" and burdened
with tension and anxiety. With this in mind the nurse needs to be alert
to the patient's communications that might indicate that his physical
needs have become secondary to his security and esteem needs.

The nurse's uniform must also be considered a part of the setting,
since she customarily wears it when she comes on duty and takes it
off when she leaves. The color white may be more symbolic of than
suitable for many present-day nursing activities, but the mystique of
white is mighty. Its aura of goodness, purity, and innocence involves
honorable social values. A sphere of sorts is drawn around such virtues,
and only the most villainous would encroach on it and insult the nurse's
"honor" by coming too close. To present a white front is to be above
reproach and too often unapproachable, since this color also symbolizes
distance and coldness. The nurse's uniform implicitly warns the patient
of the role that he is expected to play but also provides him with the
understanding that the delicate tasks carried out by the nurse "will be
performed in what has become a standardized, clinical, confidential
manner."[21]

There are many concrete variables in the setting that the nurse must
consider, such as lack of privacy and distracting noises; more important

may be the abstract generalizations that the patient may form. Although abstractions may help the individual to place the setting in some category to which he can relate, the effect on communication can be disastrous. Thus, in much the same manner the she defines her role to a patient, the nurse must also define the setting. She may do both through "professional closeness," focusing "exclusively on the interest, concerns, and need of the patient" and his family through her verbal and nonverbal communication.[22] Inherent in the concept of professional closeness is "availability," or giving the patient an opportunity to avail himself of the nurse's presence and services, to communicate as her conversational equal, and to develop further his own competencies in understanding situations, other people, and himself.[23]

NONVERBAL COMMUNICATION

Nonverbal communication is the way in which human beings influence each other without words—the way in which man expresses himself through a silent language and makes an impression on others. Nonverbal language is said to be partly taught, partly instinctive, and partly imitative. The military salute, the peal of laughter, and fasionable shoes are respective examples. Communication fundamentally involves two radically different but interdependent kinds of symbols: the deliberate impressions that one *gives* and the less deliberately controlled impressions that one *creates.* The first involves the spoken word, which is the best friend of man's public self. Verbal assertions can be skillfully used to distort, conceal, deny, disguise, and generally mask true feelings. The second set of symbols covers a wide range of human activities, from body movements to responses to the messages of others. How one listens and uses silence and the sense of touch may convey important information about the private self that is not available from conversation alone.

Both verbal and nonverbal communication may be used for deception. If the patient wishes the nurse to think highly of him or to believe that he thinks highly of her, he will take care to convey messages that will serve this purpose and be in his best interest. To sum up the matter in clichés, the patient will give a "benefit performance" to "get off on the right foot" by "going into his act" or "putting on airs." In much the same manner, "playing the role" is a part of everyday life. Thus you may have experienced the following view of some teachers:

> You can't ever let them get the upper hand on you or you're through. So I start tough. The first day I get a new class in, I let them know who's boss. . . . You've got to start off tough, then you can ease up as you go along. If you start out easy going, when you try to get tough, they'll just look at you and laugh.[24]

Similarly, "sympathetic patients in mental wards will sometimes feign bizarre symptoms so that the student nurses will not be subjected to a disappointingly sane performance."[25]

Even though an individual may take care to present himself in a calculating manner, he cannot sustain with equal guile both his speech and his actions. Having to make a choice, the individual is most likely to concentrate on the familiar and controllable aspects of communication by measuring and regulating his speech. This leaves him little time to be aware of and govern his nonverbal language. The nurse can make use of this asymmetry in communication by validating the patient's dialogue by his bodily gestures. What he does may express and reinforce what he says or contradict and belie it. Thus we say that "actions speak louder than words," since they often attest to the truth or falsity of what is said. However, motions alone may not be the message. Nonverbal communication may be accidental and incidental. A person may accidentally convey impropriety by belching and incidentally keep her knees stiffly together for propriety.

The meaning of a nonverbal clue depends on the context of the situation, as well as the person sending the message. The syntax of silent language is so complex that the use of specificity in interpretation is recommended if the intentions of the patient are to be reasonably understood. Specificity does not negate the significance of nonverbal communication. Rather it is a particular code that the nurse must decipher before meaning is given to the message.

Body language

Since man is a unified whole, his internal disposition often finds expression in both movement and nonmovement of a part or all of his body. From the following "conversation" one can see that many parts of the body reflect a feeling state: "Why is your nose out of joint?" "A certain twofaced mutual friend is such a pain in the neck that she is really getting under my skin; so, even if I'm putting my foot in my mouth, I'm so fed up I must bend your ear by getting this off my chest, or, instead of keeping my feet on the ground, I'll blow my top!" Just so, human emotions may unconsciously be translated into physical equivalents. One can observe without interviewing, but one cannot interview without observing the physical projection of an individual's emotional state in gestures, posture, gait, eating, grooming, and a host of other symbols. Again let me emphasize that body language, like all nonverbal communication, simply provides the basis for reasonable inferences, rather than precise conclusions.

When possible, the face-to-face arrangement is recommended for interviewing. People who sit opposite each other have more mutual "stimulus value" than do those who sit side by side. In communication one responds to something other than the content of the remarks, and face-to-face positions tend to produce high levels of interaction and participation when feelings or information are exchanged.[26] Thus an obvious and powerful influence on communication is the nurse's nearness, or proximity, to the individual. The side-by-side arrangement is essentially neutral but may be used if the nurse and patient turn the upper part of their bodies toward each other while sitting or look at each other periodically while walking. One can readily see that the stimulus value in the face-to-face position results from eye contact. Of all the parts of the human body "the eyes are the most important" for transmitting nonverbal information.[27]

In our culture the custom is to draw attention to the eyes through makeup, false eyelashes, contact lenses, and decorative eyeglass frames. Wearing sunglasses makes the individual less accessible to others; their removal may be a sign that the individual is becoming more receptive. For two men to look at each other for more than a brief moment is inappropriate, and a gentleman is not supposed to stare at a woman longer than a few seconds unless she gives him license with a wink, a smile, or a backward glance. Staring at people is rude. Custom dictates that, if you catch an individual staring at you, "it is his duty to look away first."[28] If he does not follow convention and continues to stare, then, whether the message is agreeable or disagreeable, you begin to question his motives. People stare at paintings, passing scenery, and animals in the zoo. To stare at people is to treat them as objects of either derision or misplaced curiosity; so one must manage not to stare at the deformed or disfigured. The potency of eye power gains more credence in everyday life by endowing certain individuals with the abilities to "look right through" and "undress" other individuals with their eyes. Eyes are an extremely important medium of communication because we rarely formulate in advance the movements of our eyes.

By manipulating the eyebrows and muscles around the eyes, a person can initiate, further, or terminate communication. "The quick look and lowering of the eyes" is body language for "I am willing to trust you."[28] To strengthen the message, one looks directly at the other's face before looking away. Sometimes the rules are hard to follow. In acknowledging another's humanness and conveying receptivity to their communications, we must avoid staring at them and yet also avoid ignoring them. Eye conventions also vary from culture to culture. In this society to project honesty you look the other person in the eyes when you converse; not to do so is to be labeled *shifty* and *untrustworthy;* yet in some cultures to "meet another's eyes with shameless boldness" is considered ill mannered.[29]

During the interview the listener usually maintains more eye contact than does the speaker. The listener's beginning to look away might indicate some doubts about the speaker's veracity or a readines to turn the attention elsewhere. Turning one's back to the speaker is as effective in terminating a conversation as is nodding or falling asleep. Eyebrows raised or lowered with a smile show agreement or interest. A frown means puzzlement or disagreement. Narrowed eyes may indicate seduction or suspicion. A furrowed brow shows intense concentration or worry. Because eye blinks can easily be counted and recorded, a better correlation may be made between a body movement and an inner emotional state. One study showed that the rate of blinks rose "when the subjects discussed topics that aroused tension or anxiety."[30] The rate also went up whenever the topic under discussion changed but fell toward the end of the topic. Eye blinking seems to be more frequent with unpleasant than with pleasant topics. When looking at pleasant or interesting materials, "as compared to neutral ones," the pupil has been found to dilate measurably.[31] Conversely, looking at distasteful or disliked material produces constriction.

The eyes have been called "the mirrors of the soul," or indices of a person's subjective state. Since eye movements are mostly unconscious, the patient's eye behavior may help the nurse to determine when an emotionally charged area is being approached. There may be even more value in the nurse's awareness that her own eye movements may unwittingly convey her feelings of repugnance when changing a dressing, doing an irrigation, or answering a call light. In decoding eye language, ours and theirs, we are better able to see ourselves.

Notice how hands may be used to orchestrate verbalizations: accentuating, punctuating, and clarifying. Generally persons from different cultures tend to speak a different body language with their hands. In Latin American countries the hands and arms play a major role in communication, and every sentence "may be accompanied by a sweeping gesture of arms and hands."[32] In contrast, we tend to use our arms and hands less frequently for gestures when conversing. Those individuals who freely and spontaneously express themselves through gestures in this culture are said to be confident extroverts. Observation of the way that a patient uses his hands may give indications of feelings and attitudes that are not being candidly verbalized. Wringing the hands, biting one's fingernails to the quick, playing with a ring, and fidgety and restless hands may be manifestations of nervousness, tension, and embarrassment. Hiding hands behind one's back and sitting on the hands symbolize shyness and insecurity. Portraits of famous men demonstrate that closed hands are a sign of masculinity, whereas American women pose with open hands to represent femininity. Gestures may be a great help in understanding the spoken word, but, in the absence of a physical impairment, the substitution of manual for verbal expression "may indicate a person's withdrawal from interpersonal involvement and a regression to a more primitive pattern of behavior."[33]

Schutz argues that the "manner in which a person holds his body indicates his mood, his background, and his present accessibility to human interchange."[34] Thus one may infer that a patient who sits with his arms and legs crossed tightly may be walling himself in and others out. By retaining this position and leaning back, the patient reinforces his opposition to interpersonal communication. This makes leaning forward in an interview a significant sign of receptivity. The body attitude of postural rigidity, although it strengthens the backbone, may suggest an uncompromising and inflexible verbal position.

The habitual visage that a patient assumes may define his sovereign temper. The postures that he adopts and emphasizes may alert the nurse to the role that the patient expects to play during the interview. Lowen thinks that a "blown-up chest is invariably a concomitant of a blown-up ego."[35] Erect and squared shoulders seem to designate determination, and a jaw that extremely protrudes "clearly indicates defiance."[36] Haughtiness may be signaled by the patient's holding his head up high and turning it to neither the left nor right. Such personal characteristics may give the nurse a hint that the patient anticipates that he "will be the one who will initiate the verbal interaction and direct its course."[37]

On the other hand, a patient may minimize his presence and physically withdraw from the setting. A bowed head, stooped shoulders, and hunched back decrease physical height with actual shrinkage in one's personal dimensions. This posture calls to mind depression, and the nurse may presume that she will have to be the one to begin verbal communication. The gait and posture of a patient on crutches hardly goes unobserved. Most nurses seem to be familiar with nonverbal communications due to physical disabilities; yet the gait and posture of an individual in a noninstitutional health care setting rarely seem significant. The nurse may better understand a patient by becoming more familiar with his habitual manner of responding without words. The patient's lapses into a different form of nonverbal communication may symbolically convey a need that he cannot readily voice. During the interview, placing both the patient's actions and words into a meaningful context is essential to therapeutic communication.

Use of touch

Since people often touch one another while gesticulating, it is difficult to clearly discriminate body language from tactile language. Although body language may not attract attention, the surest and most obvious way of decreasing social distance and making one's presence known is through touch. Touching has already been mentioned as the matrix of many nursing activities. Because touch is integral to patient care, we may view it as a generalized mode of communication that takes place in the natural course of events; but, just as all generalizations have their exceptions, many actions that we take for granted have their intricacies. If we use touch as a means of making contact with another person without foreknowledge of the possible outcomes, we may not only be anticipating a response that does not occur but will also be unprepared for what may actually materialize.

In the dominant American culture, puritanical traditions make touching shameful, for it "is equated with sexual intent, either consciously or at a less self-conscious level."[38] During the process of socialization the child soon learns from admonishments ("Stop playing with yourself! Don't touch! Keep your hands to yourself!") that it is evil to communicate with himself or others through touching; so a well-mannered individual is expected to apologize after accidentally touching a relative, friend, or stranger. Touching that is done for the sake of health, such as in a bed bath or back rub by the nurse, may be impersonally accepted, since not only are such activities prescribed but also their therapeutic effects are publicly and unabashedly described. The nurse and patient may engage in intimate physical contact without awkwardness, embarrassment, or guilt as long as they maintain a "civil inattention" to the erogenous and pleasurable aspects of the activity.

Self-identity requires that we separate ourselves conceptually from others. Moreover, given the exposed and vulnerable surface of the human body, psychologically we claim ownership of the space around us for comfort and security reasons. This need for personal distance was substantiated by Hall, who stated that an American "surrounds himself in an invisible bubble, keeping all but close personal contacts with others outside this bubble."[39] There is an implicit rule that one should present "credentials" before crossing the border of another's personal space. Handshakes are a cultural ritual to convey a "welcome sign" of intitation or a "warning sign" to keep out. The duration, firmness, and type of interlock all form parts of a message. The amount of pressure helps one to determine warmth and sincerity; a flaccid and limp handshake may mean either rejection or indifference. No interpretation of the refusal to shake an outstretched hand is needed. When the nurse reaches out to touch the patient during the interview, she needs to be aware that she, in effect, is invading the patient's personal sphere and violating the sanctity of his person. Since there is "an inward compulsion" in individuals to "possess and defend their space" as their exclusive preserve, the patient's reaction may range from righteous indignation to acute anxiety.[40] The nurse's use of touch during the interview may be more appropriate once she understands the nature of its ambiguity and complexity.

Knowing that touch has the potential to harm does not repudiate its important contributions to human well-being. Touch has been proven to be able to heal and to have other dimensions of inestimable value to the nursing process. Touch is man's first means of communication. A newborn infant primarily experiences the world through tactile contact with parents. In the process of growing up the child is encouraged to obtain information about self and the world through other sensory modalities; yet, even when grown up, the individual never seems to outgrow the need for personal contact with another human being. Rubin observed that, in situations of intense personal stress in which a person felt isolated and vulnerable, no other means of communication could compare with the comforting and quieting effects of touch.[41] Durr seems to hold essentially the same view, concluding from her study of patients convalescing from trauma or critical illness that patients perceived the nurse's use of touch as conveying security, closeness, warmth, concern, and encouragement.[42] Rapport with seriously ill patients can more readily be established through the use of touch, and findings also support the concept that, to many patients, caring is embodied in touch.[43]

Although touching seems to be the sine qua non of nursing, it is comparable to a double-edged sword. One side of the sword is said to be taboo and the other therapeutic. Since both are interlocked and capable of leaving their mark, the nurse must pay minute attention to technique, so that it will function in a balanced perspective. One side used as a separate strategy may lead to one-sided results.

The duality of the nature of touch is best expressed by Durkheim, who described the human personality as a "sacred thing"; one should not "violate or infringe its bounds, while at the same time the greatest good one can do for another is to be in communion with him."[44]

Use of silence

"What can I *do* to help achieve goals?" is a common question in the nursing process. The phase of implementation is usually formulated on the Kardex in terms of motor activities. Nursing intervention finds documentation in such functions as *turning* the patient every 2 hours, *recording* intake and output, *changing* dressings when necessary, and *taking* the pulse before giving digoxin. During the evaluative phase of the nursing process, if the nurse can not point to a specific activity and say, "This is what I did to help!" she may think that she has failed. The emphasis on doing and documenting in nursing tends to reflect the criteria of success in our action-oriented society. Thus, in communication high verbal activity, not surprisingly, replaces motor activity as the criterion of effective dialogue. Small wonder then that one of the greatest problems relating to interviewing perceived by nurses was how to handle silence.[45]

Instead of being the absence of communication, silence itself is a specific channel for transmitting and receiving messages. This awareness alone may help the nurse to accept the use of silence as a significant means of influencing and being influenced by others.

In the initial interview the patient may be reluctant to speak because of the newness of the situation, the strangeness of the nurse, self-consciousness, embarrassment, or shyness. Talking is highly individualized; some find the telephone a nuisance; yet others feel they cannot live without it. The nurse must recognize and respect individual differences in styles and tempos or responding. How else can we learn of another's nature and our own but by courtesy, care, and time? The quiet person, the individual with a language barrier or speech impediment, the elderly and persons who lack confidence in their ability to articulate, through their silences, may be communicating a need for someone to have faith in them and to help them experience success in self-expression.

Although there is no universal rule concerning how much is too much silence, silence has been postulated to be only "worthwhile" as long as it is "serving some function and is not frightening to the patient."[46] Knowing when to interject herself into the interview is largely dependent on the nurse's acuity about what is being conveyed through the silence. Sometimes the topic under discussion has been exhausted; if the patient does not begin anew, brief supportive comments or a question by the nurse may stimulate conversation in another direction. Icy silence may be an expression of anger and hostility. The "silent treatment" has been described as a destructive weapon, the "ultimate" in contempt for another person.[47] It is worse than striking a person in the face, since at least this shows recognition and strong involvement, but not to have one's presence acknowledged is one of the most hurtful things to which a human being can be subjected.

Silence may also personify emotional blocking. If the patient feels pressured to talk about a subject that he finds too painful, he may react with stony silence as a form of defiance or resistance. The nurse can intervene in a surefooted manner against resistance only when she is certain that the relationship can withstand the strain. She must also be secure enough in her own self-image and role to support the patient's silent pain without feeling that his expression is a form of personal hostility. However, the nurse may gain more if she does not pursue the conversation along the lines that evoked the initial emotion but rather supports the patient in regaining his composure and resuming[48] conversation at a level at which is most comfortable. Silence then becomes a medium of rapport that shows understanding of the patient's unreadiness to commit his feelings and emotions to verbal expression.

Successful interviewing may be largely dependent on the nurse's "will to abstain"—to hold herself back to keep from talking more than is necessary. Solitude may provide meaningful moments of reflection for both the patient and nurse. It gives them each a golden opportunity to contemplate thoughtfully what has been said and felt, to weigh alternatives, to formulate new ideas, and to gain a new perspective of the matter under discussion. It has been found that after a period of silence, if the patient was the first to speak, "the length of his responses increased."[49] Therefore a too hasty interruption by the nurse may leave significant thoughts and feelings of the patient forever unshared. That the nurse may be the first to break the silence was implied by Greenhill, who found that many patients were prevented from responding because of the maximal verbal activity of most interviewers. The nurse who feels compelled to fill every void of silence with words may often do so because of her own self-consciousness and embarrassment. Thus her need for comfort tends to take priority over concern for the patient.

Yet prolonged and frequent silences by the nurse may hinder an interview that requires verbal articulation. Although the untalkative nurse may be comfortable with her silence, this mode of communication may make the patient feel used and as though he were merely a fount of information to be drained dry. Moreover, without feedback the patient has no way of knowing whether the nurse understood what he said. Verbal patterns of student nurses have been demonstrated to correlate with therapeutic communication.[50] The *appropriate* use of verbal techniques of interviewing helped the students to focus more directly on the patient's needs and to elicit more feeling responses. The nurse who values silence highly may need to reassess the impact of her nonverbal communication on the interviewing process. Without such a reassessment she may be unable to use the creative potential of mutuality, or working together with the patient toward goals.

Although there may be no need to restate what everyone knows to be true, redundancy has merit if it reiterates the need for humility in all our human endeavors. Since it is impossible to judge accurately what is going on in another person's mind, a patient's silence during the interview does not necessarily indicate that he is mentally involved in giving the matter under discussion his undivided attention. The same expressions of rapt absorption that communicate attentiveness to the interview are not essentially different from the expressions of rapture that one projects while exploring one's fantasy world. Such is man!

Use of listening

To a patient who needs to share his thoughts and feelings, the nurse's listening may be a precious gift, requiring that the nurse use her entire being as she actively seeks to understand the diverse and subtle expressions of human beings. Through listening she creates an interpersonal situation of maximal involvement that may allow the patient to experience himself more fully and freely. In her search for meaning she observes the patient's total network of communication: his body messages, his tactile messages, his silent messages, and the messages that may be plainly or symbolically verbalized. The nurse, in turn, can communicate caring and concern for the patient by acknowledging her understanding or misunderstanding of his messages when given. Recognizing that the language of strong emotions may differ from that of conscious thought, the nurse reproaches the patient for neither his curse nor his cry.

The nurse's therapeutic self helps to strengthen the patient's ability to solve his own problems. In the depths of one's fantasy world, one does not have to make any sense; but to reach an objective, whether relief from tension or gaining information, one usually has to place one's thoughts in some semblance of order to be able to communicate immediate needs more readily to others. Giving the patient her supportive attention, the nurse communicates to him that he is not alone but with someone who will be thinking along with him to understand and help him. This kind of nursing intervention enhances self-esteem and encourages the patient to direct his energies toward reaching the discussion objectives. Serving as a "sounding board" for the patient, the nurse listens as he "tests" his thoughts by voicing them aloud. This form of interpersonal interaction often enables the patient to clarify his thinking, link up ideas, and tentatively decide what he should do and how best to do it.

Sometimes the nurse may be more therapeutic when she does *not* listen.[51] Inappropriate patient confessions may be best handled by referral or consultation. The nurse needs conscientiously to evaluate her ability to help the patient cope with the guilt and shame that is often the consequence of intense soul-searching. To do otherwise is to place the patient in jeopardy by making him bear such profoundly disturbing emotions alone. Similarly the patient who is on the verge of losing self-control through hysterical or harmful behavior may be helped to regain his composure better if the nurse actively directs and structures the interview through the use of verbal communication techniques.

Listening is hearing out loud. By paying attention to the patient's choice of words, themes of repetition and strains of omission, variations in pitch and tone of voice, crescendos of silence and assertiveness, rhythms of rapidity or slowness in speech, the nurse may obtain information that the patient may think insignificant, as well as information that he may be unable or reluctant to provide response to questioning. As the nurse listens, she may discern both harmony and discord between what she sees and hears, since the patient's personal idiosyncracies, attitudes, and feeling tones often find expression in unconscious ways of responding. Less apparent cultural differences are more likely to be observed than verbalized. How the young are socialized and the elderly and sick cared for are cultural values that the patient may view as universal norms, rather than variations that would be of interest to the nurse.

While listening, the nurse may find that timely interjections or prompting may be helpful facilitators of communication by conveying to the patient that the nurse "comprehends, is interested, and is listening carefully."[52] Spoken or unspoken encouragement should ideally neither interrupt the patient nor direct his conversation. Although brief sounds or phrases, such as *uh-huh* or *I see* and body movements, such as leaning forward in her chair and nodding her head, do not specify the scope or direction of the patient's response, such exclamations by the nurse as *oh no, how nice,* and *that's awful* are a form of wishful hearing that imposes a value judgment that biases or inhibits that patient's response.

If, for example, a father remarks to the delivery room nurse, "This is my fifth son," the nurse has no way of knowing if the father is surprised, happy, or disappointed. In much the same way, if the nurse responds with something intended to be comforting, the father has no indication as to whether the nurse is commiserating with him or subtly recommending birth control. Thus, instead of the interaction's becoming a meaningful interview, the lines of communication become entangled in misunderstanding. The nurse using listening as an interviewing technique must insist on the truth in Proverbs 18:13: "He that answereth a matter before he heareth it, it is a folly and shame unto him," for listening is the common denominator of all the other interviewing techniques and one of the basic keys to understanding.

VERBAL COMMUNICATION

Man lives in a society of symbols, and his supreme social symbol is words. Through words he forms mental images of himself and his world of people, places, and things. Words are used to express his thoughts, feelings, attitudes, and beliefs symbolically. Words are used to control his own behavior and to influence the behavior of others. Moreover, his responses to words have much in common with his responses to people and his environment. Therefore primarily through verbalization the individual communicates his definition of himself and his unique world to others.

To facilitate understanding the nurse may have to help the patient to translate the mental images of his thought and feelings into words.

Even though the nurse and the patient have the same background, the mental image they have to a word may not be exactly the same. Although believing they are talking about the same thing, they may in reality be talking about something quite different. The word *trip* gives testimony to the manner in which differences in mental images can produce misunderstanding. Should a nurse say to a patient, "I heard you had some trip," he will define *trip* according to the images that he has formed of the word from speaking, reading, writing, and listening. Depending on the patient's past experiences the nurse's fairly innocuous statement could convey interest or insult. Did the nurse think that he stumbled and fell? Did she think that he traveled to another city? Does she possibly think that he experimented with a drug and "flew" without leaving his room and without benefit of technology! Tending to reflect the rapid, widespread changes in society, words often capriciously change meanings and are therefore best interpreted in accordance with the company they keep.

Communication between persons from different cultures may be hindered by a lack of sufficient understanding, so that one statement may simultaneously convey different messages. One of the messages is transmitted *explicitly*, or with the precise meaning of the sentence, whereas the other message is communicated by *implication*, or the meaning that the speaker wishes to convey at the moment. In our culture the question, "Why don't you drop in some time?" is not a request for a visit. If it were a true invitation, a specific date and hour would be set. However, someone from a different background may take the "hostess" at "her word" and create an embarrassing situation for all concerned. That Americans can say one thing and at the same time mean another may be baffling to someone unfamiliar with the way that we use words. Many remarks are no more than noncommittal social amenities: "Nice weather we're having" or "Hi, how are you?" These remarks are made in passing, and the speaker neither expects to be detained to listen to a confirming weather report nor indicates a willingness to listen to another's biography. More information has to be communicated either verbally or nonverbally to make the statements personally relevant. However, in interviewing, the use of some social pleasantries may be necessary to put the patient at ease and to establish a climate for more meaningful communication.

All this is to emphasize that words are the work of the individual's mind and that the nurse must not assume that in verbal exchange there is also an exchange of equivalencies of meanings. Without the knowledge of the nurse or patient, pseudocommunication may occur because one or the other failed to interpret the message as intended. One way in which the meeting of minds may be effectively accomplished is through the skillful and purposive use of questions. Skillfully put questions can lead to understanding far more "persuasively than the most logical argument,"[53] for to ask not is to guess a lot!

Use of questions

Essential to therapeutic communication is the use of questions. To make a nursing diagnosis, during the interview the nurse seeks answers to three key questions involving three goals: "What is the patient's problem?""What does the problem mean to him?" and "How is he adapting to the situation?"[54] Keeping her objectives in mind helps the nurse to formulate purposeful and effective subquestions and to limit her inquiry to what is pertinent to achieving her objectives. The questions that she uses to encourage appropriate levels of self-disclosure are meant clearly and simply to elicit information that can be used to develop a realistic and personalized plan of care. Therefore the nurse focuses on the immediate needs that the patient may be communicating nonverbally and verbally. Even though all patients have needs, they do not have the same problems in either expressing or meeting their needs. Thus the nurse may reach her goals more readily in some interviews than in others. Regardless of the nature of the interview, questions that probe and seek to expose hidden motivations have no place in therapeutic communication. A wound that is probed may heal, a mind that is probed may be irreparably wounded. To be able to identify and meet a basic human need the nurse does not need to delve into the motives and drives underlying that need. Although one patient may hunger for affection because he was brought up in an orphanage, another may hunger for affection because of frequent moves with his family to different neighborhoods. So diversified and complex are human motivations that false assumptions are more usual than unusual.

In the process of gathering data the nurse organizes and formulates questions that will clearly communicate to the patient the goals of the interview. Knowing what kind of information is wanted may stimulate his thinking toward the discussion objective.

Yet the patient's participation in the interview does not mean that he will give *only* information that is logically relevant to the discussion objectives. To ask a patient (who will be called *Mr. Clay* in all the subsequent examples) if the prescribed medication relieved his chest pain the night before may not elicit either a yes, no, or maybe but a lengthy discourse, "The Effects of Hospital Personnel, Bed and Bedding, and Snoring Roommates on the Biologic Rhythms of Paying Patients." Although this may be irritating to the nurse, she must try to be generous in spirit and not become too impatient, since people do not meander off into irrelevancy accidentally. In one's mental processes, both emo-

tions and reason insist on expression; when emotions become sufficiently strong, whatever the motivation, they cannot be blocked by reason. The patient who introduces illogical irrelevancies into the conversation has not necessarily been inattentive to the discussion or misunderstood the question: the subject at hand may not be as "emotionally
relevant" as his need to release anxiety, to be in touch with another,
and to reassert his identity through the display of intellect, virtues, or
grievances.[55] Unless the patient is able to fulfill some of these needs
through his illogical digressions, he may not be disposed to answer the
nurse's logical and relevant questions. Listening to a patient's irrelevancies may increase the nurse's understanding of him and acceptance
of his need to transmit in conversation something other than pure
thought. Although the nurse may not have gained the specific information that she sought, by establishing a relationship that is emotionally
satisfying to the patient, she may find that future interviews are more
conducive to the meeting of minds.

   Types of questions: open, closed, and leading. The interrogative mode of communication, or questioning, is said to be "one of civilized man's most
effective tactics for getting the other fellow on the defensive."[56] When
we ask questions, we, in effect, are requesting that another individual
interrupt mental free play or concentration, attend to our ideas, and
supply us with information on demand. Whether the answer is readily
available or has to be worked out, to respond, the other person's thinking must be directed to the topics that we select. If the previously mentioned prerequisites for therapeutic communication are met, the nurse
will not ask or demand of the patient more than she is willing to give.

   Such interrogatives ask for factual information: *what, which,
where, when,* and *who.* In reference to Mr. Clay the nurse, if given
the opportunity, might have interpersed the conversation with questions
such as the following:

   · What seems to aggravate the pain?
   · Which position do you find most comfortable?
   · Where is the pain acute?
   · When did it start?
   · Whom did you report it to?

   The use of the interrogative *why* or its variations puts the patient
on the defensive and is not recommended as a therapeutic technique.
The "psychologic why" implies an expectation of the patient to provide
insights into the causes for or purposes of his behavior, which may be
unknown to him. Even if he can answer the *why,* he may defend himself
by evoking the Fifth Amendment verbally or nonverbally. It probably
would have been useless to ask Mr. Clay:

   · Why are you avoiding the discussion of your chest pain?

Or variations of the same question:
- How is it that you seem indifferent to discussing your chest pain?
- What keeps you from answering questions about your chest pain?

To answer such questions, Mr. Clay would need to have a deep under-standing of the manner in which the subconscious human psyche af-fects personality needs. We know that he has a great need for human contact, but knowing why this is so is irrelevant.

Generally the how and what questions are more difficult to answer with a *yes* or *no* and thus encourage more descriptive patient responses. "How did your chest pain last night differ from the night before, Mr. Clay?" and similarly, "What do you think happened last night to make it worse?" tend to stimulate greater cognitive activity and verbal com-munication.

The manner in which the nurse uses interrogatives to preface key words in the question may be seen to influence or direct the patient's replies. Thus questions are differentiated into two general categories—*open* or *closed*—depending on the degree to which they structure an-swers. An open or broad line of questioning does not influence the direc-tion of the patient's responses, and his answers are open-ended ranges of possibilities. Closed questions ask for specific data and provide limited choices of patient response.

Through use of the nondirective technique the patient is encouraged to express in his own way his ideas on a particular topic and structures the answer in his own mind as he chooses. Because more involvement is required to express ideas concerning the position that one takes, the patient's response to a broad question tends to convey more feeling and information than do the answers to clinical questions.

To continue the analogy with Mr. Clay, should the nurse inquire, "What happened last night to disturb your sleep?" and "How do you think we can help you to be more comfortable at night?" she gives the pa-tient an opportunity to present in greater detail his personal point of view.

Often the nondirective technique makes use of the open-ended, or incomplete, statement. The nurse begins such sentences by repeating information that Mr. Clay may already have given: "And then after you received the medication. . ." or "You were saying about the pain. . . " The raised inflection at the end of the sentence invites the patient to furnish his own ideas in completing the statement and to focus in greater depth on the topic under discussion.

In contrast, to answer a closed question the patient supplies specific facts without deviation from the topic. Since the nurse structures the question, it requires less thinking for the patient to answer; for example, "Is the pain on the right or left?" gives Mr. Clay two choices. Likewise, "Do you have any pain now?" merely requires a *yes* or *no* and does not readily allow for the expression of his reactions to his discomfort.

The nurse may find both types of questions helpful in achieving the goals of the interview, but *how* she uses the questions is as important as the formulation of a particular one, since the patient is mentally reacting to both the tone and content of the question. If the nurse and patient are strangers, he may be on guard, wondering what the nurse is like and whether they will be able to talk to each other without difficulty. Her first words to him create an impression that tends to answer his unspoken question. An anxious patient may be made to feel more comfortable if the nurse begins with closed questions that not only help to delineate his area of interest rather quickly but also ask for information that he experiences success in giving.

Perceiving the nurse's interest in him, he feels more confident and safe. With the reduction in anxiety he may become more expressive in an atmosphere in which he thinks that he will be understood.

Although the closed question can be answered briefly, often the patient feels impelled to qualify his answer spontaneously. To return again to Mr. Clay and the initial question by the nurse, "Did the prescribed medication relieve your pain last night?" he might have replied, "Yes, *but* I still couldn't rest because. . ." Generally after the use of such conjunctions the nurse's "third ear" is needed, since this is often the most significant part of the patient's message from his point of view.

Closed questions may also be the most appropriate for eliciting clear-cut and precise information, such as the patient's name, age, and religion. On the other hand, a patient who is negative and reluctant to communicate verbally may be more responsive to questions that he can answer in a free and individualistic manner before he is ready to divulge specific information to the nurse.

Thus the effectiveness of any question should be evaluated in terms of the patient's response. Both the closed and open-ended questions can convey concern for and interest in the patient. However, the thoughtful use of the nondirective technique gives the patient the initiative to disclose himself, voice his doubts and fears, and tell of his problem in his own way. Because the nurse follows the patient's leads and responds to his ideas, the use of the open-ended question may be the most helpful to the nurse in getting to know the patient as a person—his thoughts, feelings, and wishes. From such knowledge may come a better understanding of the nature of his problem, of him, and of herself.

Leading questions are closed and not only suggest the direction of the patient's responses but also let the patient know what the nurse expects the reply to be. By guiding the patient's response to a preselected answer, the nurse is likely to get an emotional reaction, rather than a thoughtful rejoinder. Such questions as "You know we're doing everything to help you, Mr. Clay, don't you?" or "Don't you know that you're getting the very best of care, Mr. Clay?" lead the patient to choose the answer that the nurse has recommended. "Would you say that you are being treated differently than other patients, Mr. Clay?" might be a more subtle expression of the same question. The question challenges the patient to affirm the nurse's efforts appreciatively without further ceremony. Even though the nurse is really questioning his integrity, he may be too embarrassed, shy, and eager to please or simply not wish to defend himself by giving an explanation. However, the raised eyebrow, blinking of his eyes, clenched jaw, or tense posture may well express the patient's negative reactions to the appeal to his emotions, rather than to his intellect. Although the nurse has a right not to like an answer that the patient gives, the patient also has the right to answer without intimidation the questions that she asks.

Clarifying techniques

Understanding depends on clear communication, which is aided by the nurse's verifying with the patient *her* perceptions of his messages. By requesting feedback on the accuracy of her listening and observations the nurse avoids the implication of being critical of the manner in which the patient expresses himself. The use of clarifying techniques assists both the nurse and patient in identifying major differences in their frames of reference and gives them both the opportunity to clear up misperceptions before they aggregate into misunderstandings. When the nurse requests the patient to elaborate on or clarify his vague or ambiguous messages, she is communicating to him that she very much wants to understand him and is providing him with a means to understand her. Orlando believes that, if the nurse subscribes to the uniqueness of each individual's experience, she must learn "responsive discipline, the discipline which phrases or formulates her perceptions or thoughts by questioning and wondering about the meaning of them to the patient."[57] This kind of exploration, in turn, enables the patient to respond by either validating or clarifying the nurse's impressions of him and his impressions of her.

Use of paraphrasing. For clarity the nurse might restate in newer and fewer words the basic content of a patient's message. Using simple, precise, and culturally relevant terms, the nurse may confirm without delay her interpretation of the patient's previous message before the interview proceeds. Prefacing her statements with such phrases as "I am not sure I understand . . ." or "In other words, you seem to be saying . . ." the nurse helps the patient to form a clearer perception of what he has said while at the same time giving a sense of coherence to what may be a bewildering mass of details. After the nurse has paraphrased, she must validate the accuracy and helpfulness of her restatement in promoting understanding. The patient may confirm or deny her perceptions through nonverbal cues or by directly responding to a question by the nurse, such as "Was I correct in saying that . . . ?" As a consequence the patient is made aware of the fact that the nurse is thinking about and with him. This translation of the nurse's commitment into words helps him to feel understood.

Use of reflection. Using reflection, the nurse mirrors for the patient his overt and covert messages. Thus the nurse may use this technique to echo content, as well as feelings. In a manner different from paraphrasing, when the content of the patient's communication is being reflected, the nurse repeats the same key words that the patient has just spoken. As a corollary, should Mr. Clay remark, "My life has been full of pain," the nurse may gain additional information by reflecting, "Your life has been full of pain. . . ." The purpose is to stimulate further elaboration of significant areas that are being vaguely or ambiguously expressed by the patient. However, too frequent and indiscriminate use of reflection might convey to the patient that the nurse is disinterested and inattentive. Parroting and mimicry can make nondirective techniques ludicrous and block communication.

Another key to understanding the patient is reflecting the feelings that his messages communicate. The nurse describes briefly to the patient the apparent meaning to her of the feeling tones of his verbal and nonverbal behavior. By way of example, to reflect to Mr. Clay his feelings of anger the nurse might begin, "You say that as if you were very angry," "You seem to be feeling angry," or "You look angry." By incorporating her observation into such statements and sharing them with the patient in a manner that conveys acceptance, the nurse helps to bring the patient's feelings into his awareness and encourages his ownership of them. This may serve to emphasize to the patient that the goals of the interview relate to both his emotional and physical needs and that the informational content of his messages is not preeminent. Perceiving that the nurse's concern may parallel his own, the patient may more spontaneously express and clarify his feelings.

When the patient-nurse relationship is a trusting one, the nurse may facilitate understanding through the use of the techniques that reflect her impression of the patient's total communicative experience. With sincerity and tact the nurse may use the technique of confronting the patient with the disparities between his explicit and implicit messages. The nurse shares her assessment of the patient's behavior by such statements as "You say that medication relieved your chest pain, Mr. Clay; yet I notice that you are clutching your chest." Confrontation has to be used with caution because in effect it is "catching a patient in a lie." A variation on the same nurse's observation might be "You say that the medication did not relieve your pain, Mr. Clay; yet I notice that you are breathing normally." If the patient accepts his inconsistencies as a "little white lie," he may further explore with the nurse the accuracy or inaccuracy of her impressions. If he is threatened, he may feel prodded into denying the nurse's total impression without further ado, for people seem to be more disturbed by revealing half a truth than by concealing the whole truth.

Use of summarizing. Mutual understanding may be promoted when the nurse feeds back to the patient the general substance of the interview as she sees it. This technique unifies a number of pieces of information into main themes of content and feelings. By highlighting the most significant data, the nurse can determine with the patient what progress they have made and also again whether the information obtained is accurate before making future plans. This cooperative patient-nurse interaction gives the patient the feeling of contributing toward the resolution of his problem and reaffirms his sense of worth.

To avoid forming inaccurate patient concepts, the use of clarifying techniques offers the nurse many flexible options. When integrated with the other interviewing skills, they assist the nurse and patient in gaining and maintaining compatible frames of reference. If all the keys to understanding are used with humanity rather than mechanically, human accord is more likely to be achieved.

The search for meaning is a difficult task. The nurse receives messages from the patient in one form and has to translate these new and complex phenomena into simpler and more familiar alternate forms. This search for meaning is called *compassionate thinking*. "If we are successful, we call it understanding."[58]

REFERENCES

1. Miller, G.: A psychology of communication, New York, 1975, Basic Books, Inc., Publishers, p. 46.
2. Chorover, S.: Big brother and psychotechnology, Psychology Today, p. 54, Oct., 1973.
3. Greenhill, M.: Interviewing with a purpose, American Journal of Nursing **56:**1259, 1956.
4. Haney, W.: Communication and organizational behavior, Chicago, 1967, Richard D. Irwin, Inc., p. 88.
5. Skipper, J., Tagliacozzo, D., and Mauksch, H.: What communication means to patients, American Journal of Nursing **64:**101-103, 1964.
6. Siegel, N.: What is a therapeutic community? Nursing Outlook **12:**49-51, 1964.
7. Goffman, E.: The presentation of self in everyday life, New York, 1959, Doubleday & Co., Inc., p. 33.
8. Whiting, J.: Patient's needs, nurses' needs, and the healing process, American Journal of Nursing **59:**661-665, 1959.
9. Jackson, J.: Communication is important, American Journal of Nursing **59:**90-93, 1959.
10. Ruesch, J.: Therapeutic communication, New York, W. W. Norton & Co., Inc., 1961, p. 462.
11. Goldin, P., and Russell, B.: Therapeutic communication, American Journal of Nursing **60:**1928-1929, 1960.
12. Aiken, L., and Aiden, J.: A systematic approach to the evaluation of interpersonal relationships, American Journal of Nursing **73:**865, 1973.
13. Zunin, L., and Zunin, N.: Contact: the first four minutes, Los Angeles, 1972, Nash Publishing Corporation, p. 15.
14. Ibid., p. 6.
15. Jourard, S.: How well do you know your patients? American Journal of Nursing **59:**1568-1571, 1959.

16. Thornton, G.: The effects of wearing glasses upon the judgement of personality traits, Journal of Applied Psychology **28**:203-207, 1944.
17. Byrne, D.: Interpersonal attraction and attitude similarity, Journal of Abnormal Sociology and Psychology **62**:713-715, 1961.
18. Matson, F., and Montagu, A., editors: Human dialogue, New York, 1957, The Free Press, p. 159.
19. Garrett, A.: Interviewing: its principles and methods, New York, 1972, Family Association of America, p. 72.
20. Minckley, G.: Space and place in patient care, American Journal of Nursing **68**:511-516.
21. Goffman, op. cit., p. 26.
22. Peplau, H.: Professional closeness, Nursing Forum **4**:343-359, 1969.
23. Schmidt, J.: Availability: a concept of nursing practice, American Journal of Nursing **72**:1086-1089, 1972.
24. Becker, H.: Social class variations in the teacher-pupil relationship, Journal of Educational Sociology **25**:459, 1963.
25. Goffman, op. cit., p. 18.
26. Steinzor, B.: The spatial factor in face-to-face discussion groups, Journal of Abnormal Social Psychology **45**:552-555, 1950.
27. Fast, J.: Body language, New York, 1974, M. Evans & Co., Inc., p. 122.
28. Ibid., p. 139.
29. Ibid., p. 132.
30. Spiegel, J., and Machotke, P.: Messages of the body, New York, 1974, The Free Press, p. 66.
31. Berelson, Bernard, and Steiner, G.: Human behavior, New York, 1964, Harcourt Brace Jovanovich, Inc., p. 103.
32. Fast, op. cit., p. 118.
33. Hein, E.: Communication in nursing practice, Boston, 1973, Little, Brown & Co., p. 164.
34. Schutz, W.: Joy: expanding human awareness, New York, 1967, Grove Press, Inc., p. 36.
35. Lowen, A.: Physical dynamics of character structure, New York, 1959, Grune & Stratton, Inc., p. 90.
36. Ibid., p. 94.
37. Goffman, op. cit., p. 24.
38. Jourard, S., and Rubin, J.: Self-disclosure and touching: a study of two modes of interpersonal encounters and their inter-relation, Journal of Humanistic Psychology **8**:39-48, 1968.
39. Hall, E.: Hidden dimension, New York, Doubleday & Co., Inc., pp. 112-113.
40. Ardrey, R.: The territorial imperative, New York, 1966, Atheneum Publishers, p. 3.
41. Rubin, R.: Maternal touch, Nursing Outlook **11**:828-831, 1963.
42. Durr, C.: Hands that help: but how? Nursing Research **10**:392-400, 1971.
43. McGorkle, R.: Effects of touch on seriously ill patients, Nursing Research **23**:125-132, 1974.
44. Durkheim, E.: Sociology and philosophy, translated by D. F. Pocock, New York, 1953, The Free Press, p. 37.
45. Ushvendra, K.: Verbal responses of nurses to patients in emotional-laden situations in public health nursing, Nursing Research **16**:365-368, 1967.
46. Schulman, E.: Intervention in human services, St. Louis, 1974, The C. V. Mosby Co., p. 123.
47. Wahlous, S.: Family communication, New York, 1974, Macmillan Publishing Co., Inc., p. 147.
48. Schulman, op. cit., p. 125.
49. Richardson, S., Dohrenwend, B., and Klein, D.: Interviewing: its forms and functions, New York, 1965, Basic Books, Inc., Publishers, p. 257.
50. Johnson, B.: The relationship between verbal patterns of nursing students and therapeutic effectiveness, Nursing Research **13**:339-341, 1964.
51. Mahoney, S.: The art of helping people effectively, New York, 1967, Association Press, p. 122.
52. Richardson, Dohrenwend, and Klein, op. cit., p. 199.
53. Nirenberg, J.: Getting through to people, Englewood Cliffs, N.J., 1963, Prentice-Hall, Inc., p. 116.
54. Prange, R., and Martin, H.: Aids to understanding patients, Nursing Outlook **62**:98-100, 1962.
55. Nirenberg, op. cit., p. 98.
56. Miller, op. cit., p. 125.
57. Orlando, I.: The dynamic nurse-patient relationship, New York, 1961, G. P. Putnam's Sons, p. 41.
58. Miller, op. cit., p. 49.

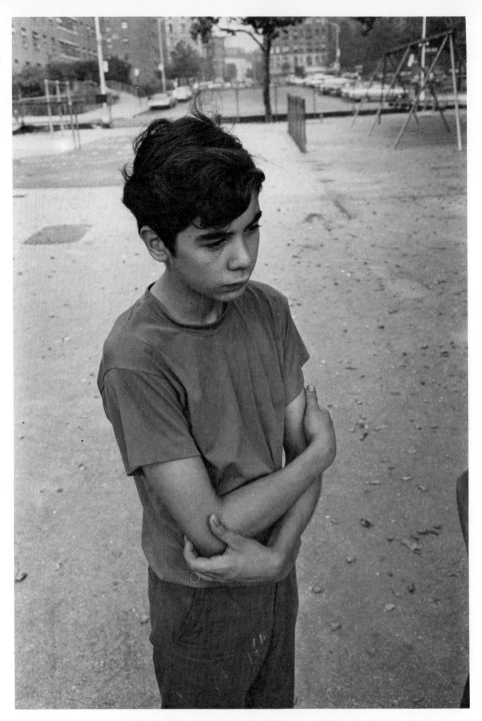

Life is a process of continuous change. The stress of rapid, unrelenting change may damage the mind as disease damages the body and cause the individual to drift *inward* to deal with the stress by avoidance. The affective responses to stress—anxiety and depression—heighten self-concern, cutting the individual off from spontaneous human experiences. He may wall himself in . . . and all others out. (Photograph by James Carroll, Editorial Photocolor Archives.)

CHAPTER 4

Characteristic behaviors of those needing help

OVERVIEW

The pace of life has quickened, and anything, pleasant or unpleasant, that speeds up the tempo of life causes an increase in stress, "the wear and tear exerted upon the body."[1] The body responds to stress of any kind with a unified defense mechanism that can facilitate adaptation to damage as well as cause it. Thus, on the physiologic level, man's immunologic defenses ward off invading microorganisms. Psychologically man's mental defenses protect him from anything contrary to his desires. Socioculturally the individual's religion, family, or other forms of group solidarity may be powerful allayers of stress.

Although these adjustive mechanisms seem impressive, they are nonetheless limited in preventing adverse personality responses to stress. The family and the church, once impregnable social institutions, have made their concessions to change by altering their functions and seem not to provide as much strength and support as before. This occurs at a time when a swiftly changing social order has caused an accretion in the rate and sources of stress; yet in this culture a person is expected to exert intelligent control over inner conflicts while coping with the strain of disagreeable situations. In other words, in the absence of organic disease, man's adjustment-response mechanisms should continue to prevent maladaptive behavior. However, when stress is acute or accumulates, man resorts to whatever resources will best serve to mitigate the threats to his sense of integrity and wholeness. Personality decompensation is often incompatible with self-preservation, and the prototypes of his protective responses are anxious and depressive behavior. Depending on the interplay of such factors as health status, motivation, personal experience, social setting, and interpersonal relationships, the individual's anxious and depressive adjustments may range from normal to pathologic.

ANXIETY

Some say that man is born anxious. Rank was perhaps one of the most articulate proponents of the view that anxious moments in later life are but re-creations of the "initial anxiety" experienced during the "trauma of birth."[2] In comparison, Tillich[3] concluded that all anxiety derives basically from man's conscious or unconscious acknowledgment that his "nonbeing" inheres in the simple act of "being." Combining both points of view is the conclusion that man comes into the world anxious and is made more so by the knowledge of his own impermanence. Thus human beings seem destined to experience in life many unpleasant sensations of apprehension and dread that are vague as to cause. In truth the stress of modern living has made such an impact on this saga of human destiny that anxiety now is said to have "come of age." The contagious and "free-floating" nature of this malady is democratic, and no one seems to be spared. Throughout the life cycle, covert feelings of insecurity and unease are being pressured into more overt expressions. However, unlike fear, the causes of anxiety are nonspecific. In effect, man exists in an era that threatens his sense of stability; yet his anxious reactions shed no light on that which is threatening.

Regardless of this inconsistency, anxiety is analogous to pain and just as significant in alerting man to possible danger. When he is confronted with real or imagined danger from the unknown or untried, his anxiety activates an alarm system of varying degrees of intensity. Physiologically his body prepares him for "fight or flight" and body processes that facilitate adaptation are mobilized.[4] The degree of this energized reaction is personalized, for one person's minor concern may be another's major problem. In much the same way, visible manifestations of anxiety tend to be multiple. Included in this array are muscular tension; insomnia; digestive disturbances; elevations of pulse, respiration, and blood pressure; frequent urination; trembling; increased perspiration; easy fatigability; and changes in the pattern of speech.

Psychologically, mild or "normal" anxiety increases alertness and stimulates self-improvement as well as goads the individual into improved performance. In brief, mild anxiety may be conducive to learning because it scares people "into their wits." On the other hand, moderate anxiety narrows the person's perceptual field, and details essential to the solution of a problem may be ignored. Inattention to meaningful factors impairs one's ability to abstract and draw realistic conclusions. Anxiety is often aroused by the individual's own unacceptable thoughts and impulses rather than by a realistic external cause. Neurotic anxiety results when chronic worry is the only reaction to unidentified problems. Such anxiety sometimes causes signs of cardiorespiratory distress, which may convince the person that death is imminent. When anxiety reaches this level of severity, the minutiae in a problematic situation have become disproportionate to the whole. This loss of objectivity and scattering of ideas increases the possibility of distortion and irrational behavior. Phobic reactions and panic are attempts to escape from unbearable situations. In the latter the patient's flight may terminate in either agitated or withdrawn behavior.

Defenses

Man's prodigious mind makes him a virtuoso in defending himself from anxiety. Anxiety is painful, and he will go to great lengths to avoid and conceal it from himself and others. Some of the mechanisms he uses occur so frequently in everyday behavior that they have been classified. When used in moderation, these defense mechanisms are healthy means of containing one's anxiety and instinctual drives, as well as preserving a positive sense of self. In carrying out these functions, all the mechanisms, which are largely unconscious, contain elements of self-deception.

The boundaries that distinguish one defense mechanism from another are not clearly marked. The mechanisms overlap, and more than one may be operant at the same time. Explaining the manner in which each supports and protects the ego may highlight their usefulness.

Denial. Denial is a means of defending the ego against anxiety by the conscious refusal to admit the very existence of painful emotions, memories, or experiences. It is fundamental to all the other mechanisms. This mental pretense that all is well minimizes the threat to our sense of security and continuity; yet there would be no need to use this mechanism to avoid facing reality if at some level of awareness the truth were not already "known." This may be of import in the care of the terminally ill patient.

Rationalization. All of us like to think that our behavior is sensible and based on creditable motives. We justify our conduct to ourselves and others in such a way that it *seems* reasonable, whereas the true reasons for our behavior are kept from our conscious awareness. Behavior that is plausible arouses less anxiety and maintains self-esteem. So, when a student nurse does something without the instructor's approval, the latter often interprets such behavior as inability to work under supervision due to underlying hostility toward authority. However, when instructors overstep their bounds in a given situation, they refer to their action as a manifestation of autonomy, self-direction, and initiative!

Projection. Projection is a form of rationalization that protects us from negative self-image through the psychic process of assigning our undesirable characteristics to others. Suppose that a nurse has a tendency to be harsh and unkind; it would be traumatic to her ego if this basic disposition were recognized. However, self-deceit would rather easily convince the nurse that a patient's chief mission in life is to make her miserable. Since the patient is cruel and insensitive, he deserves any harsh treatment that he gets. He is entirely at fault; she herself is blameless.

Identification. Identification is the opposite of projection. This mechanism is operant when someone who suffers a loss of self-esteem tries to alleviate the resultant anxiety and a gnawing sense of worthlessness by association with an organization, institution, group, or individual perceived as having great worth. Identification can help a person to feel secure at crucial times. The hospitalized patient who receives visits and remembrances from his lodge brothers feels more positively regarded, and this sense of self is a valuable asset in his battle against illness. Identification is a normal part of the process of growth and acculturation. Children integrate into their own egos the qualities of those to whom they feel a strong emotional attachment. Remember, however, that these qualities may be social or antisocial.

Introjection. Introjection is the integrating of ideas and ideals external to oneself into the core of one's own being. This mechanism is closely related to identification but has the potential for causing considerable difficulty when it intensifies and perpetuates grief. If a deceased person was the primary source of gratification of a mourner's needs, the mourner might attempt to manage the resultant anxiety by incorporating some of the characteristics of the deceased. By living in the way that the other person might have lived, the survivor eventually may forfeit identity.

Displacement, or substitution. "Don't take it out on me!" is another person's defense against the defense mechanism of displacement, which is the redirection of hostile impulses from one who is strong enough to retaliate to a safer target. This pecking order is often evident when staff nurses express their displeasure over their assignments by being critical of student nurses. Such diversionary tactics of projecting hostile impulses prevent their introjection, which could lead to self-hate or strong feelings of self-devaluation. Of extreme relevance is the implication that nurses need to be more tolerant of the patient's ventilation of hostility and in fact should encourage its expression in a reasonably acceptable manner because negative self-evaluations often precede acts of self-destruction. Displacement is a fascinating mechanism; not only introjected but also projected hostility can furnish sufficient drive to end one's life. Real or imagined grievances are settled with planned punishment: by committing suicide the individual hopes to make the person "responsible" suffer with protracted feelings of self-recrimination and guilt.

Reaction formation. Some ideas admitted to consciousness would be disastrous to one's self-image; thus there is often the tendency to adopt the opposite attitude and try to keep a measure of control over the anxiety-producing thoughts and feelings. This form of denial, however, is not always successful. For example, take the person who could never be a nurse because she just could not stand the sight of blood or to see people suffer. Yet, while eating a rare steak, she will regale one with the macabre details of the latest film depicting the catastrophic destruction of half the human race. Although the irony of the situation may escape her, fires and accidents rarely do.

Repression and suppression. Repression is what accounts for the myth of the "good old days." Although painful memories may be gone, the emotions attached to them are not. These powerful emotions may generate disturbing internal conflicts, convert into physical symptoms, or emerge as compulsive behavior. Compulsive routines unconsciously ensure that the forbidden acts symbolized by the ritual will not be carried out. Repression is an automatic maneuver that is beyond one's control. It differs from *suppression,* which is a premeditated attempt to put something out of one's mind and maintain self-control. Repression may be operating when we find that for no reason a certain patient's voice "rubs us the wrong way." Trying not to feel that way and refraining from telling him to shut up is suppression. Each is a means of dealing with disturbing thoughts and the anxiety they engender.

Sublimation and compensation. Unacceptable thoughts and impulses may be concealed and controlled through socially approved substitutions. When successful, this mechanism reduces the anxiety associated with self-rejection and leads to creative and constructive behavior. Frustrated sexual impulses may find expression in romantic lyrics or a satisfying hobby, such as sculpture. Another form of substitution is the strenuous effort to deal with anxiety by excelling in one area as a means of compensating for a weakness in another. A corollary example would be the student nurse whose performance in the clinical area is minimally satisfactory but who studies so diligently that her classroom performance is beyond reproach.

An interesting form of compensation is termed *overcompensation* in which individuals deny their weaknesses by attempting to excel in their weakest areas to avoid a sense of inferiority. A short teenager may make up for lack of stature by becoming a gang leader and issuing orders to others.

Regression. Man's ego tries to make more tolerable the discomfort of threatening situations by reverting to behavior that once brought a sense of security or pleasure. Student nurses away from home for the first time often line their beds with stuffed animals. Although the rationalization for this behavior is that the animals are cute and decorative, they are really nothing more than reassurances that nothing has changed. Most persons lapse into this kind of behavior now and then. Stamping feet and slamming doors are called *letting off steam* but are really adult temper tantrums. Excessive reliance on this mechanism as a means of resolving problems and dealing with frustration results in diminished self-esteem. The anxiety underlying this self-belittlement can reach such proportions that a major psychiatric disorder may result.

Summary. In summary, let me emphasize that stress increases the use of the mental devices described and that these unconscious reactions protect the individual from excessive anxiety and the loss of self-esteem. This temporary moratorium on destructive emotions helps to sustain us as we search for more realistic and mature ways of handling stress. The defenses provide us with a salutary character armor in the face of adversity and for the misfortunes that must be faced.

Nursing intervention

Communication with the anxious patient may be more therapeutic if the following variables are considered. One of the first is the nurse's recognition of anxiety in herself, as well as in the patient, so that her behavior will not be disadvantageous to either. Anxiety is infectious, and the nurse's anxiety may increase the patient's own beyond his level of tolerance. The primary goals of nursing intervention are to reduce the level of anxiety in the patient, so that he is better able to resolve his problems and to prevent maladjustive behavior. Because of the diverse responses to anxiety the nurse needs to communicate to the patient what his verbal and nonverbal behavior seem to be indicating and that his behavior is understandable and she would like to know more about it to help him.

If from her observations the nurse concludes that the patient's anxiety level is not increased by verbalizing what he is experiencing, she should help him to identify the anxiety as such. By giving a specific name to his unpleasant sensations, the reality of the patient's pain is shared, and what is perceived as realistic is often handled in a less bewildering manner.

Anxiety is an anticipatory emotional response to the new; thus anticipatory guidance may not only alleviate anxiety but also prevent its emergence. Nurse-patient exploration of the precipitating factor is recommended, even though the real reason for the anxiety remains unknown. Once a probably cause is discerned, the provocation can be related to its effect; thus seeing the relationships in a problem facilitates its solution.

To return to Tillich's theory that all anxiety has as its genesis the fear of becoming nothing, the anxiety engendered from man's feelings of emptiness—that he is "nobody"—may be of such magnitude that his second automatic protective mechanism, depression, will stealthily erupt as his major defense.

DEPRESSION
Overview

The age of anxiety, with its accelerated courses of cultural and social change, keeps the stream of life storm tossed and driven. Just when the individual thinks that the day's currents of change have been weathered, on the horizon are seen the gathering clouds forecasting change in the future. As a rational animal, man believes in the efficacy of his intellectual processes in facing and dealing with reality. His values and beliefs embody his deepest commitment to the way that human life should be lived. They are the cognitive maps that he uses in setting and working toward goals. The conscious and unconscious standards that man sets for himself give his life a sense of direction, meaning and purpose. Not only do his values remind him of where he is going but also of who he is, and they provide the emotional ballast needed to navigate the sea of change.

All life's experiences—every human relationship, thought, and action —"registers in the brain's emotional center as pleasurable" and life supporting or "painful" and life negating.[5] The brain keeps a tally. Man estimates his personal worth by the sum of his successes and failures. He experiences this estimate of himself constantly, and how he regards himself is crucial to the nature of his human experiences.

Rationality implies that man characteristically behaves in ways that are beneficial to his welfare and survival. The rewards of making good choices are pleasure, a sense of control over one's existence, and a belief that, in such a "benevolent" world, one's aspirations are attainable. To the extent that the decisions he makes give sustenance to his life, the individual feels self-reliant and self-assured. This sense of mastery does not mean that he will not make errors but that he feels adequate in evaluating and handling his mistakes. Suppose, however, that the individual experiences repeated difficulty in achieving goals and is generally unsuccessful in meeting his basic human needs. In this competitive, achievement-oriented society a person who fails is likely to feel like a failure. Although "to err is human," this does not make the psychic pain more bearable, for it is against the policy of the brain to forgive. Instead a warning is given to the individual that his behavior is not beneficial, that he is in "improper psychologic condition," and that his "relationship to reality is wrong."[6] Viewing his cognitive processes with skepticism and himself as inept and ineffectual in relating to reality, the person may abandon the captaincy of his fate and retreat from a world filled with "malevolence." Feelings of self-devaluation are reinforced by the whole world's love for a "winner" and society's decree that the "best man always wins!" Our system's social rewards have made winning everything, although we still go on saying, "It's how you play the game." When self-appraisal correlates with accomplishments more than self-knowledge, the individal becomes extremely vulnerable to crises in self-esteem.

Present-day man has many choices; when formerly one's choices may have been limited to one clear-cut course of action, today there are many viable alternatives. Moreover, the evidence of what is appropriate or inappropriate is continuously fluctuating. In this pluralistic society the moral signposts that once charted the "ideal" course have become ambiguous and arbitrary. Heterogeneity in life-styles has made homogeneity of values obsolete. Since there is no exclusivity of belief or absolutes of true and false, "all is relative," and what is relative may also be contradictory. Thus a person may believe that "anything worth doing is worth doing well" and yet be unable to reconcile this credo with the feelings of frustration, anger, and low morale that result from the dreary passivity of assembly line tasks. Boredom and the bomb threaten to overtake him.

The surging tides of social change rock every boat. In an attempt to stay "enlightened," individuals must address themselves more assiduously than ever to the task of discriminating between what is suitable or unsuitable before they can respond with integrity and intelligence to their surroundings. The continuous flow of new and diverse information must be evaluated and previously held attitudes about the self and the nature of the world reevaluated. Cognitive self-confidence is difficult to maintain when solutions to one's problems are only tentative and any decisions that one makes are subject to revision.

Society mandates that man adapt, adjust, and be flexible. Admirable though the courage of one's convictions may be, "inflexibility" conflicts with the other "virtues," and a value held as desirable may have to be jettisoned if it makes the individual impervious to change. To be of firm character and open to change is a contradiction of human nature. Although conflicting moral standards and values can be verbalized and rationalized, they cannot be integrated into the subconscious. Thus modern man is in a perpetual state of disquietude. His actions must be in accord not only with his contemporaries but also with the verities of his conscience, for the "standing orders" of the superego are inexorable and unyielding. A friend of the traditional past and a foe of the future and change, the conscience is much less concerned with actual social practice than with the "principle of the thing." If the nurse believes that abortions are wrong except to save the life of the mother, she cannot care for such a patient without a great deal of emotional trauma. Similarly the nurse's knowledge that estrogen in the "pill" induces premature "epiphyseal closure," or advanced bone age in teenagers, may so compromise her preventive health value that working in a family-planning clinic may leave her guilt-ridden.[7] Profound values made dispensable produce intense psychologic anguish. Even minor infractions do not go exactly unnoticed. Substituting cheesecake for a carrot stick on a reducing diet may initiate a process of self-reproach, as well as digestion. Should man fail to make amends, the feelings of frustration, resentment, and guilt will sabotage his sense of worth and self-respect.

Since there is no value judgment more important to man and no factor more decisive to his psychologic security and well-being than the estimate he makes of himself, small wonder that depression is the most important consequence of diminished self-esteem.[8]

Terminology

Depression is a troublesome reality and a troublesome concept that describes different realities. It is a synonym for *transient feeling states, persistent mood disorders,* and *specific psychiatric syndromes.* As a transient feeling state, depression colors the world blue for most persons at one time or another during life's enterprise, since whatever the experiences of self-realization, there will be heightened moments of sadness because of internal conflicts, environmental setbacks, and acts of parting from people, places, positions, and possessions. Bleak periods of mourning for actual or impending interpersonal losses are also a part of living. Generally, however, man's cognitive functioning is essentially unimpaired, and neither the "blues" nor grief becomes interminable. In time the gloom lifts and individuals reaffirm themselves in continued hopes and aspirations; but, like all human responses, depression involves degrees of depth, duration, and intensity. When depression has such tenacity that the individual loses the perspective of reality and the totality of existence is colored enduringly black, the mood is labeled a *psychiatric symptom.* Such is the nature of this despair that feelings of autonomy capitulate to those of helplessness and hopelessness and the person's usual adaptive capacities are stilled by a sense of futility. Depression can progress insidiously. Should man no longer relate to the world through reason but instead through delusions and hallucinations, his depressive reaction constitutes one of the dramatically apparent psychiatric syndromes with names such as involutional melancholia and manic-depressive psychosis. Thus the concept of depression seems to become more definitive when it is evaluated in terms of its effects on the individual's reality testing.

The terms *exogenous* and *endogenous* categorize depression as to causes. When depression seems to be a reaction to identifiable precipitating factors in the environment, it is referred to as *exogenous.* Despondency that occurs as a result of internal factors, such as a change in the brain level of norepinephrine, is called *endogenous.*[9]

Further differentiation of depressive patient behavior is made in terms of *retarded* or *agitated* motor functioning. For both types of patients, the scenario of life is regarded pessimistically. In short, the retarded depressed person expresses psychic pain through a decline in activity level. In contrast, the agitated despairing individual communicates anguish through stereotyped movements, such as pacing back and forth over the same territory.

It is noteworthy that the word *depression* is common to lay and medical terminology. This everyday usage may make it easy for the nurse to misinterpret its nature, and the ramifications of depression may be seriously underestimated. However, depression can be a major mental maneuver against the anxiety engendered by self-devaluation, and any defense mechanism that persistently covers up can also be costly. Vigilant protection of a beleaguered ego requires a tremendous amount of energy and deprives man of the full use of his mental capabilities for problem solving. Because his process of data gathering tends to rely more on emotions than intellect, the nurse's data-gathering process necessitates astuteness in observation and communication. Moreover, since there tend to be fewer opportunities for the patient to satisfy his needs for reassurance, appreciation, and a sense of dignity within readily accessible supporting groups, the blows to his ego may be devastating. Regardless of the classification and categories of depression, the person truly hurts, and the patient-nurse relationship must ensure that experiences of quiet desperation will not be endured alone.

Communication

Overview. Because of its manifold relationship to a variety of human complaints, depression, like syphilis, is a great imitator. Depression may precede an illness such as cancer and also accompany the common cold.[10] Physical illness and depression may simulate each other. Almost invariably the depressed patient presents a physical sign or symptom that seems to be immune to the most vigorous medical investigation and treatment. In truth, there are "gut feelings and reactions"; Rice has observed that the gastrointestinal tract is the site of choice for symptoms of depression.[11] Conversely, the patient who offers no complaints may be feeling so dejected that he thinks it is useless to do so. Depression is an integral component of most human situations that threaten the individual's usual state of homeostasis. Depression may be masked by obesity or be a consequence of attaining a svelte figure. Depressive reactions are a part of illnesses that involve changes in one's life and of recovery that involves adjustments to life. Such is the perniciousness of despair that it is believed to cause "more human suffering that any other single disease, mental or physical."[12] Regardless of her professional field, the nurse will not fail to encounter this affliction in one of its many guises.

Traditionally in many nursing curricula the care of the "medical" or "surgical" patient is taught in the general hospital wards and clinics, and instruction in the care of the "psychiatric" patient takes place in a separate wing or building. Most often the patients with the major depressive disorders in psychiatry seem to have radically different nursing diagnoses from the low-spirited patients on the general ward. Somehow in the transfer of learning, *depression* undergoes a metamorphosis in meaning, and what was despairing behavior on the psychiatric unit becomes "good" behavior in the general patient population. Fortified by a belief that abnormal behavior is always bizarre, the nurse may find pleasure in caring for the good patient because she scarcely knows he is there. However, despite the noticeable difference in degree of psychomotor retardation, patients in both settings share a common lowered emotional tone of "sadness, helplessness, and hopelessness."[13] Just so, these solemn and silent communications of depression must not go unheard or unheeded.

Nonverbal communication. To a great extent, recent changes in the individual's customary level of function may reliably communicate some of the salient features of depression. Although no one patient is likely to manifest all the behavioral changes, the presence of even *one* of the characteristics warrants further investigation. Nonverbally the patient's "organ dialect" and muscular tonus speak for the man within, and the classic modes of this silent language find expression in the following areas.

Sleep patterns. Compatible with depression is an increased need for sleep, difficulty in falling asleep, or awakening very early in the morning. Early morning awakening is said to be the most common change. Typically the patient feels worst in the mornings and gradually improves as the hours pass. This diurnal variation in intensity of symptoms is "one of the most clearly diagnostic signs of depressive disorders."[14] Thus, repeated assessment at different times of day is vital to making an accurate nursing diagnosis.

Weight. Notice that the depressed individual may overeat and gain weight. However, anorexia and unplanned weight loss is the most distinctive result. The amount of this loss may be a measure of the degree of the patient's self-abasement and feelings of being unworthy to exist. Eating sparingly causes his facial and other body muscles to sag and makes him appear older than his chronologic age.

Appearance. The patient simply stops treating himself well and neglects his normal hygienic practices. His unkempt appearance may reflect the depths of his self-contempt. His demeanor is morose with a downward turning of the corners of his mouth and a furrowing of his brow. From time to time he may indicate his state of utter forlornness with sighs of resignation. A valuable clue to the recognition of depression may be the nurse's own feelings of sadness when she is in the patinet's presence, although no words have passed between them. However, she must not be unwittingly drawn into his depressive state because in that case, instead of intervening to alleviate his distress, she might well become a part of it.

Body processes. The throes of despondency often coincide with a general pattern of deceleration in the individual's normal physiologic and physical processes. Gastrointestinal slowdown may be recorded in the nurse's notes as constipation. The graph of vital signs will show a decline: "the pulse rate is slower than normal, blood pressure reduced and respiratory rate retarded."[15] The female patient's menstrual cycle may be out of phase, with amenorrhea, or absence of menses, the predominant disturbance. Although some patients expend energy in flurries of unproductive activities, most often the depressed patient uses his energy to sustain the impression of inertia and prefers to sit or lie down for a good part of the day. Little enthusiasm is shown for activities that were once considered enjoyable or activities, such as reading, that require concentration. General vitality is depleted: gestures are few and less animated and walking is slowed to a dragging gait. As a consequence of the decreased muscle tonus, lowered energy level, and inattentiveness to anything in the environment other than himself, accident proneness may also be a sign of depression in the patient.

Interpersonal relationships. Despair causes the patient to restrict his sphere of concerns and commitments. Emotional retrenchment, with its limited expectations of self, is preferable to the insecurity that may result from others' expectations. Withdrawal is an expression of social impotence and disenfranchisement in human affairs. The desire for social interaction is anesthetized by depression. Since there is no "I can," thus there is no "I must," and the challenge of interpersonal contact is averted and avoided. His emotions are economized to support his internal conflicts, and a lowered libido makes his sexuality passive. In time his interpersonal life recedes.

Depression is a process of erosion. Unchecked it may lead to an incurable disease. Wordlessly the patient may be entreating the nurse for succor and support.

Verbal communication. The healing process may begin once the nurse validates her visual observations with verbal interchange. The product of human thought, in depression, is impoverished. The choice of words is meager, and they are denuded of imagery and stripped to literalness. There is a short attention span for thoughts unrelated to the patient's despair. This is protective: by limiting the number of ideas to be considered, the individual automatically excludes those which may add to his pain. Verbal communication is dominated by monosyllables delivered in a slow, soft monotone. Captive to his psychic chaos, the patient exhumes his past and tearfully dissects it under a microscope of guilt. Remorse and self-condemnation form a pattern of circular reasoning: "No matter what I do, nothing ever turns out right! Therefore I am good for nothing. Since I am good for nothing, there is nothing I can ever do right." There is a parsimony of symbols representative of present or future strategies; the patient is convinced that he is destined to live out his life in abject misery. The variant forms of self-flagellation become self-propagating, and the patient seems unable to extricate himself from his mental morass. Wails of self-denigration are present to some extent in many depressive conversations and as such are some of its "most impressive" dynamics.[16]

Yet there are instances when depression may not cause a melodramatic disruption of the individual's habitual style of conversing. Many patients can and do continue to speak in a manner that does not directly convey their despair. In this culture one tends not to divulge concern for one's mental health spontaneously. Still, we all have our "off moments"; none of us is "all there" all the time. However, being stigmatized as emotionally unwell poses more of a threat to man's ego than do his feelings of disconsolation. Thus the person may not realize that he needs help that can be provided. He rationalizes his lament so that it conforms to the work ethic, and his symptoms suggest overperformance rather than substandard performance of his social responsibilities; so the common, everyday depression of frustrated man in a demanding world is embodied in complaints of general weariness.

Unrecognized depression clouds all aspects of the nursing process, and care given the patient has more shadow than substance. In other words, *not* to be alert to the communications of depression is to let the individual suffer until surcease from mental torment is found in spontaneous remission or death. Of extreme importance is the fact that depressive feelings are often self-limiting and rarely representative of a lifelong emotional pattern.[17] Thus a significant key to understanding depression is a fairly recent change in the patient's general approach to life. People who know the patient intimately can expedite the nursing diagnosis. Such observations as the patient is "not himself" or has "somehow changed" helps the nurse to assess the difference between the patient's present and past methods of functioning. The despondent patient anticipates no relief. In varying degrees his mental processes are incapacitated by the conviction that his despair is interminable. Solutions to most of life's problems have yet to be perfected, and rational choices may indeed be imperfect. Solutions often demand a challenging search. Disarmed by life, the depressed individual may be unable to meet this challenge and come eventually to the one solution that is unequivocal. For such a person the illness of depression may prove to be fatal.

Suicide. Every 24 minutes someone in the United States who has evaluated existence and found it wanting ends it.[18] This blight on humanity may be even greater than statistics report. Better to let cultural taboos simplify and classify the matter under "respectable" accidents than to confront the possibility that, for some, death has more redeeming value than life. Although acts of self-destruction are related to other causes, such as disorientation from delusions, toxic fevers, and untoward response to drugs, they are most often associated with depression. Still, some people may willingly take their lives in the absence of depression. Soldiers have been known to die for the "common good," and martyrs throughout history have sacrificed their lives for ideologies that they held sacred. Even when depression is evident, the danger of suicide is not always proportionate to its degree. A patient with a terminal illness may be profoundly despondent and although on the verge of death, not actively seek it. Even though the major complication of depression is self-destruction, there are other significant factors that potentiate the risk of suicide. These may or may not occur together with recognizable depression and can appear separately or together. Only total team participation in ongoing observations make them relevant. There is no disputing the fact that the priority of nursing intervention is preventing an affliction for which there is no cure. Thus the nurse should also manifestly consider the following criteria in the assessment of suicidal risk:

1. Hostility, projected or introjected, seems basic to all suicidal patterns. In fact, suicide is impossible without it. Hostility, "with its aggressive component, provides the biological driving force" that is a prerequisite for acts of self-destruction.[19] Thus the presence or absence of a wholesome aggressive drive in the patient may indicate an increased need for vigilance. The withdrawn patient who displays no recognizable signs of hostility needs as much observation as does the individual whose outward expressions of hostility become more intense or cease. In this regard, any changes in the patient's behavior, for better or worse, may be premonitory indications of suicide. Beware of the patient who becomes too social too soon and whose recuperative powers seem too remarkable. Many suicides have been reported to occur within a few days after the patient has apparently improved, since the energy used to sustain his state of relative inertia is now freed to commit the act.[20]

2. Suicide is seldom the impulsive act that it seems. When the patient begins to have suicidal thoughts, the idea of self-destruction so terrorizes him that typically he will hint at the act to come. Although his verbal messages may be direct, indirect, or coded, the majority of suicidal patients are ambivalent. They wish to be rid of their problems and yet survive. Nothing is more direct than "I am going to end it all!" and indirectly the patient may convey his lethal inclinations by simply bidding the nurse farewell as she goes off duty. A subtly coded message

may be from the patient's "friend," who wants to know the procedure for leaving one's eyes to an eye bank. Through these communications the patient is trying to notify others of his need to be saved from himself. If the message is missed and help is not forthcoming, such a notice may well be his epitaph.

3. Nonverbally the patient may communicate a tentative commitment to death by making a "practice run." No matter how halfheartedly run the race or how feeble the suicidal gesture, the event must be judged as serious. True, his behavior may be attention getting, manipulative, and cruelly controlling, but all individuals tend to use the psychologic ploy that best serves their needs. Retaliatory anger or contempt further demean the patient, and perhaps this is one of the reasons that the mortality rate of subsequent attempts at self-injury is so high.[20]

4. Although an overwhelming number of persons who take their lives are depressed, many are not "mad," or psychotic. In contrast to the addictive or alcoholic patient who is chronically on the verge of suicide, individuals with stable personalities may be acutely suicidal. The patient scheduled for or recovering from mutilating surgery may find the status of the sick role so incongruent with his values of a meaningful life that he cooly calculates to end it. One of the most painful realizations is that life has lost all meaning, without which there is little to be concerned or care about. Then, too, treatment and treatment failure may be a concomitant to suicide. Severe and unrelieved respiratory distress, a complication of epidemic proportions in heart and lung diseases, is more often associated with suicide than are other chronic illnesses or malignancies.[21] In these instances, organic deterioration, rather than mental incapacitation, may be a prodromal sign of suicide.

5. Psychoanalytic theory avers that man has an innate wish for death. Existing social phenomena have been found to give impetus to his natural propensity for self-extinction. Apropos are two of Durkheim's classifications of suicides—"egoistic and anomic."[22] Egoistic suicides result from the lack of strong group ties, and anomic suicide may occur when the standards of the group to which an individual belongs no longer give life a sense of regularity. In the latter type of suicide, rather than face the challenge of change, the person severs the ties to life. However, the more prevalent of the two is egoistic suicide. Meaningful interpersonal relationships are the very essence of mental health. Disruptions of significant relationships by marital conflict, separation, divorce, ruined careers, and death may constitute emotional emergencies. Unshared stress may make an individual a high risk for suicide. Persons who have to rely on only their own strength may become too exhausted to continue the struggle. The nurse needs to be especially sensitive to the fact that man's sense of aloneness may be more starkly realized during festive holidays, which symbolize warm interpersonal

contact; and the anniversary dates of upsetting events in prior years may be commemorated alone by self-annihilation.

6. Beginnings, as well as endings, seem to activate the death instinct. Beginnings are promising times of renewal, and, with the quickened pace of human endeavors, hopes and dreams are also reawakened. Springtime, the beginning of the week, and daybreak seem particularly provocative. With fatalism the person may conclude that to extinguish all hope is far better than to face more hopeless days. In much the same manner, lonely weekends in the hospital may set the stage for suicide.[23] The reduction in staff also reduces human interaction and involvement, which may accentuate the patient's feelings of estrangement and uselessness.

Nursing intervention. In this society the pursuit of happiness is, in reality, a waxing and waning of many experiences, and some of life's experiences are colored by the murky hues of gloom and doom. Humanitarian considerations require that the question of suicide be faced with candor. It is not only a tragic loss of life but also a lifelong tragedy to the survivors. Since the majority of presuicidal persons have entertained suicidal thoughts, the nurse's questioning about this possibility is not premature or ill considered. Presupposing that the patient will react negatively to a thoughtful and concerned remark is to deny the patient's need for effective nursing intervention. Suicide is a painful malady that cannot be prevented by avoidance. The nurse need not fear that she can implant a lethal idea in a patient's mind simply by discussing it; the patient has his own ideas one way or the other. Although some individuals will not be deterred from ending their lives, the overwhelming majority of patients are "looking for a rescuer to serve as an alter ego at a time when their own ego functions are severely impaired."[24] However, this alter ego must withstand the test of the patient's ambivalence. The nurse may hear, "Go away, I don't need any help," simultaneously with the patient's nonverbal solicitations for help. The purpose of this behavior is twofold: to mask his own feelings of inadequacy and to unmask any insincerity in the nurse's offer of help.

The nurse, rather than remove herself from the situation, must enter into it and focus her inquiry on the patient's suicidal plans. Remarkably, many individuals tend to disclose their suicidal plans truthfully to someone who they believe can help them reenter the mainstream of humanity. Concrete suicidal plans relative to method, place, and time are ominous, especially if the method is lethal and readily available. Such a patient should not be left unattended or unprotected. On the other hand, the individual whose plans are vague, and the one who selects a method known to be limited in its success may not be in imminent danger. Still, continuous observation is mandatory.

Consultations are vital to the success of the nursing process, and the nurse should indulge her dependency needs and consult. She cannot support the patient if she is overwhelmed by her own anxiety from the sense of urgency that seems inherent in the assessment of suicidal potential. Consultations need not always be formal, and false alarms do not warrant apologies. Better to act when the flames seem to be smoldering than to have to react to a conflagration.

Nursing measures that enhance self-esteem diminish depression. Activities in which the patient can successfully gratify some of his needs and experience a sense of accomplishment are beneficial to his self-concept. The physical expenditure of energy during the performance of such activities will help him to discharge some of his anger, and, once this has abated, he may feel more encouraged to experience his own possibilities in moving toward the resolution of his problems and to face the anxiety that results when conflicts are no longer repressed.

Hope opposes despair, and no problem can be surmounted without it. Hope is neither false cheer nor forced optimism, but rather a nurturing faith. Nurturance communicates to the patient the nurse's belief that he has inestimable value and that the nursing process will be of value to him. Having this motivation for her subsequent actions, the nurse may make it more apparent to the patient that the nature of his condition is known, that, although his symptoms are uncomfortable, they are not uncommon, and that he can be helped. Hope is also faith; and feelings of faith can be shared. The nurse's faith that the patient can make it, as others have, may cause him to believe that he can.

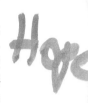

DIFFERENCES BETWEEN ANXIETY AND DEPRESSION

Anxiety and depression are both liaisons of living, and sometimes distinguishing between the two is difficult. Moreover, the two responses may coexist in the same patient in normal and pathologic degrees. One who defends his ego against anxiety with depression, in turn, may become overwhelmingly apprehensive about the depths of his despair. The following comparative observations may be helpful in differentiating these two entities.[17]

The anxious patient tends to verbalize his emotional difficulties with relative ease and is often eager to do so. In contrast, the depressed individual tends to avoid conversation and volunteers little, if any, elaborative information. Generally the depressed patient is difficult to get started talking about his symptoms, and the anxious patient is hard to stop. The anxious patient is animated in the early part of the day and may tire toward evening, but the depressed individual typically feels worse in the morning and somewhat better later in the day.

Although the external environment holds no interest for the despondent patient, the one who is anxious may enjoy listening to the radio, writing a letter, or socializing in the patients' lounge. This tendency to socialization also finds expression in dietary habits, and he may look forward to meals and enjoy food from home. Except in rare cases of anorexia nervosa, the anxious patient tends to sustain his weight. Depression is usually characterized by a loss of appetite and weight. However, some persons manifest their anxiety or depression by eating constantly and thus gain weight.

Anxiety and depression have opposite effects on the lower gastrointestinal tract: anxiety causes diarrhea and depression constipation. Another significant variation is manifested in the vital signs. The anxious person's pulse, respiration, and blood pressure tend to be elevated, but with depression these vital signs are lowered. Because of a general tendency to hyperactivity in anxious patients, tranquilizers are the drugs of choice in their treatment. Conversely, depression is generally relieved by antidepressants and enhanced by tranquilizers.

In the manners thus stated, the anxious individual anticipates the future; the depressive one reverts to the past. Although bereft of a compass, the anxious patient plunges into the stream of life, whereas the depressed patient remains ashore buried in resignation.

ANXIETY, DEPRESSION, AND THE STAGES OF MAN

All the world has been claimed to be a stage, and the drama of human life as critiqued by Erikson is played out in an orderly and progressive sequence of eight distinctive acts.[25] Therefore each phase of the life cycle will be vulnerable to anxiety and depression, since to be human is to be anxious and anxiety often leaves depression in its wake. From infancy to old age the interactional roles that man must play can be suffused with these emotions and his subsequent performances affected by them. The successful staging of each act seems to be largely contingent on the nature of the individual's social relationships. These personal relationships not only lay the foundation for human behavior but also are props to support the individual in negotiating specific developmental tasks. When the structure of social encounters no longer is a bulwark, the individual's chief safeguards may be the scaffolds of anxiety and depression. Problems become manifold, and the potential for ego disruption becomes multiple. The scope of these phenomena and the depths of anxiety and depression may be better envisaged when people and events are placed in the larger narrative of life.

Infancy: trust vs. mistrust

During the early months of life the needs of the helpless child can be satisfied only through the ministrations of others. A well-handled or loved infant develops a sense of trust and security, but an emotionally deprived one may form a pattern of anxiety and insecurity. Sullivan believed that "anxiety about anything in the mother induces anxiety

in the infant"[26] and the formation of a depressive perspective. Regardless of the sources of anxiety the mistrustful and insecure infant may
develop a specific syndrome of withdrawal and debilitation and look very
much like a depressed little old man. Can infants take their own lives?
In the literal sense of the word, yes, for, in spite of adequate medical
care, babies have been known to wither away to death from marasmus,
or extreme emaciation.[27]

Early childhood: autonomy vs. shame

Around the second year of life the well-adjusted child develops an
autonomous, yet rebellious, self-will, expressed by no! Growth and maturation enables "holding on" or "letting go" during the process of toilet
training. The limited self-control that is beginning to be experienced
enhances the sense of self. If there is not too much conflict with the
parents, the child emerges from this stage self-confident and proud.
Harsh treatment, however, creates anxiety and shame. This self-opinion
may be manifested in despondence that takes the form of "hyperactivity," instead of the more adult "motor retardation."[28] Thus the nurse
may observe temper tantrums, sleep disturbances, fretfulness, gri-
maces, tics, blinking, stuttering, and sniffles. Also during this stage the
child learns to blush with shame and embarrassment. The child may
mask inner sadness through the physical display of extreme rage. Extraordinary as it may seem, Brussel and Irwin state that head bangers
"seem bent on suicide and removing themselves bodily from a milieu
that brings them psychic pain."[29]

Play age: initiative vs. guilt

The preschooler takes the initiative in using increased skills in locomotion and communication to broaden the world through imagination,
play, curious questions, and fantasy. Fantasies help to fulfill wishes
and dissipate hostility. However, since they gain ascendance at the same
time as does the superego, fantasies can provoke extreme anxiety. Those
concerning Oedipal desires are not only frightening in themselves but
also because they may be found out. Since thoughts at this age are believed to be synonymous with the actual deed, much guilt and shame
may ensue. When abetted by the parents' love and their moral standards
of conduct, the child learns to redirect unacceptable impulses and work
with others toward a given goal. The pride that comes from a sense
of accomplishment makes the child, even though small, feel of equal
worth to others. On the other hand, severe discipline and a lack of affection inhibit the child's initiative in exploring new skills and instill the
concept of *"bad"* and *"worthless" me.* The subsequent hatred of the
punishing person is punished in turn by the conscience with feelings
of anxiety and guilt. The depressive reaction that follows is apparent

in interpersonal relationships. Instead of having confident interactions, the child seems unable to cope and sadly hangs on the fringes of groups. The energy required to keep unacceptable feelings repressed leaves little enthusiasm, "initiative or spontaneity, and less friendly feelings toward others."[30] That suicidal ideation occurs at this age has been documented by the case of a preschool boy who sought to take his life by "pouring boiling water over himself and burning himself with a gas heater."[31]

School age: industry vs. inferiority

Erikson believes that, if the developmental tasks of the first three phases have been mastered, the child enters this stage with sufficient ego strength to interact with a variety of people, accept instructions, and relate to peers according to formal rules. Industriousness is evident in the desire to know, to learn, and to produce. Concomitant to industriousness is the desire to gain recognition and pleasure from productivity. Productivity in this sense ranges from the completion of a homework assignment to rubbing sticks together on a camping trip to start a fire. The child who feels unloved and rejected enters this stage with feelings of inferiority and inadequacy. The intolerable anxiety created by these feelings may cause underachievement. This unhappy state may also be revealed in physical complaints of stomachaches and headaches. A negative self-concept is expressed in misconduct, from petty thievery and truancy to arson. During this stage, depressive feelings give rise to accident proneness, which must be considered as conscious or unconscious expression of a "wish to die."[32] Of relevance are the "increased numbers of children age 9-13" who are making frankly suicidal attempts.[33] Although the ingestion of pills seems to be the mode of choice, hangings and jumping from high places are by no means rare.

Adolescence: identity vs. identity diffusion

The fifth stage concerns neither a child nor an adult but an individual who cannot answer the question, "Who am I?" The body, now undergoing tumultuous changes, becomes unfamiliar, and the appearance of secondary sex characteristics tend to create self-consciousness. The onrush of sexuality may cause guilt over sexual yearnings, and any "deformity," such as a case of acne, can cause great anxiety. One task is to give up dependence on adults and to form new attachments independently. The need to experiment with various roles may conflict with the wishes of parents. The anxiety and mood changes engendered are normal developmental responses to the "loss," or giving up, of old relationships for new ones. In addition to these familiar expressions of depression, the adolescent may mask deep feelings of moroseness with restlessness, boredom, difficulty in concentration, and a rapid loss of interest in his usual activities.[33] Scholastic difficulties may lead to dropping out of school and experimenting with such self-administered antidepressants as drugs, alcohol, and sexual promiscuity. Prolonged delinquent behavior may induce feelings of self-reproach and self-devaluation, and the ensuing depression is often combated by identification with a subculture.

Courtship is another activity in which the adolescent seeks to achieve a positive self-concept. So total can be the immersion in this experience that rejection becomes a catastrophe, which reactivates the early pain of separation from the parents, and this pain potentiates anguish from being unable to achieve a longed-for closeness with another. In adolescence a broken romance is the "most common precipitating factor" in acts of self-destruction.[34]

Anything that threatens the attainment of an identity during this stage will also threaten existence. Thus the inability to identify with family members or peers may be a more valid explanation of why accidents are the number-one cause of mortality, rather than the popular assumption that the teenager is asserting identity. In particular the question must be raised as to why car accidents occur so frequently in late adolescence, the time that one's sensory, physical, and psychomotor functioning is at its peak.

To speculate further, teenage pregnancies may be antidepressant maneuvers. What better antidote to feelings of emptiness than to become "filled up" through conception? Without the support of any statistical analysis, the postulate that adolescent pregnancies confer some immunity to suicide is not too farfetched.

Young adulthood: intimacy vs. isolation

The young adult who has achieved a sense of identity may for the first time be in touch with inner feelings, resources, and range of capabilities and possibilities. From this beginning knowledge of self comes the ability to develop genuinely intimate relationships with others. Unacceptable adjustments in this stage may lead to a life-style of sporadic and superficial relationships. This lack of intimate emotional involvement with another is a kind of self-imposed isolation that has anxiety and depression as its constant companions. In light of the other developmental tasks of this stage—career planning, establishing strong group bonds in friendship and marriage, and building a family—the isolated person is more vulnerable to feelings of anomie and suicide.

All the tasks of this stage seem to involve roles of reorientation, new expectations, and often a new kind of existence. These can present significant hazards to even the most well-adjusted individual's sense of equilibrium. Thus exogenous, or reactive, depression is the common emotional response to unrealizable goals, career problems, and disrupted interpersonal relationships.

High standards of achievement may contribute to the increased incidence of depression. Formal education beyond the high school level is becoming a must. These greater expectations create more opportunities for frustration and disappointment. Contrary to what might be expected, most depression and suicides in college students do not occur at examination time but "earlier in the school year as the student finds himself unable to live up to his expectations."[35] However, having a degree is no guarantee that the individual will get a job in a chosen field. Raised sights must now be lowered to make a living, and employment problems make a major contribution to the incidence of reactive depression.

Couples often enter into one-to-one relationships with stardust in their eyes. Although love is blind, intimacy confers on each participant a degree in ophthalmology, and minor faults often become magnified to major defects if one or both expected pure, unadulterated bliss. When fantasies fade, feelings of frustration and failure may be laid bare. The resultant anxiety, self-recriminations, and depression may be relieved or intensified by separation.

Part of the couple's plans for "getting ahead" may be parenthood, but 9 months may be insufficient time for some to "grow up" and become "responsible." The depression that many mothers experience after the birth of a baby is so common that it merits its own classification. Although postpartum depression has a physiologic basis, the mother's unacceptable or ambivalent feelings about the infant are significant variables in her anxiety-depression reaction. Mothers need to be helped to accept the fact that "bundles of joy" can also be bundles of pain.

In recent years the young adult has become increasingly associated with the use of nonprescription antidepressants. Although drugs such as alcohol and marijuana may lift the depression temporarily, dependence on their use generally creates more problems, and the need to tranquilize oneself increases.

The incidence of depression in the young seems to be rising at such an alarming rate that Mead predicts that likely "every American adult will suffer in his lifetime at least one depression severe enough to warrant medical attention."[36] Unfortunately, too many of these episodes currently end in reported and unreported suicides.

Adulthood: generativity vs. self-absorption

The mature adult expresses generosity toward his fellow man by giving of himself creatively and productively in the role of marriage partner, parent, and co-worker. This expanded ego interest grows out of a need to be needed by others and to take a place in society. The person makes a social contribution through active concern for guiding the next generation and making the world a better place for them. The opposite of generativity is regression to a childlike level of self-absorption. The individual, like a true egocentric, indulges himself as if he were his own or another's only child. Interpersonal relationships become impoverished and stagnated in discontentment by the self-centeredness of the participants.

According to Erikson's description of generativity, the middle years can be the most comfortable of all the stages, but in this culture they may also be ravaged by anxiety and depression. At the height of a financial and occupational position, the person must now be concerned about younger competition, stepping down, and retirement. He has already been where he is going, and depression may succeed success. Much may have been demanded in its achievement—loss of sleep, ulcers, and strained or ruined interpersonal relationships. Acute anxiety and depression may be the answer to the question, "Is this all there is?"

Physiologic events cause a decline in vitality; the now childless home seems lonely and empty. There is increased pessimism and hypochondriasis concerning somatic complaints as the names of contemporaries begin to appear in the obiturary columns with disquieting frequency. Parents may begin to show the effects of physical and mental deterioration, and their illness or death makes one's own much more foreseeable. Although more common in women than in men, a form of depression called *involutional melancholia* may appear. For both comes the realization that youth is gone, and one's self-image has to change if one is to continue to feel worthy. The woman whose self-concept derived from the status and role of motherhood may find difficulty in creating a compensatory social identity, and the void may become filled with depression. Tacit acknowledgment by society is given to the man's frenzied attempts to escape his feelings of demoralization, and his antidepressant maneuvers are referred to as his *second childhood.*

Although the incidence of suicides is rapidly increasing in the younger age groups, "more than half of all suicides are by persons over 45 years old."[37] During the middle years the combined psychologic and biologic stresses arouse a kind of fearful anxiety, and the hopeless depression that follows overwhelms the self-preservative tendencies.

Old age: integrity vs. despair[38]

In Erikson's later works the final stage of man deals with old age. If the problems in the seven previous states have been successfully resolved, the individual attains an emotional integration and views his life as meaningful and well spent. Having no regrets over the past, he has more potential for accepting what lies ahead with equanimity. The lack of ego integrity, or a self-concept with which one is content, signifies despair and regret for what might have been. Time is running out with none left to begin anew, and the feeling that one has not yet lived causes fear of facing death.

Positive self-regard and a sense of status and meaning are vital in all the phases of the life cycle; but perhaps they are even more crucial in the later years, since this is the time they are most threatened. Conditions that normally increase suicidal potential are maximized and seem concomitant with aging. Longevity brings losses—loss of loved ones, health, status, income, flexibility, and capacity to cope with change. In addition, there is the lack of hope for a full recovery from illness, an awareness of the eventuality of death, and loneliness from the neglect or indifference of others. Older people can die from loneliness; they commit suicide gradually by "simply giving up on themselves."[39]

Some of the signs and symptoms of depression may be easily attributed to the aging process itself: a slowing of speech and actions, poor appetite, constipation, loss of weight, and difficulty in concentration. It is important to notice whether these are recent changes and if they are accompanied by feelings of worthlessness and hopelessness. Depression is said to be involved in 80% of the suicidal attempts by people over the age of 60, and these attempts are rarely idle gestures.[40]

• • •

Man becomes human through the process of interacting with others and may also be dehumanized in the same way. Thus anxiety and depression can be totally unrelated to organic conditions but relate simply to the condition of being human. The more we understand about the behavior of humankind in general, the more humanely we behave toward persons who happen to become patients. When we are sensitive to the reasons for behavior, we are less likely to condemn it. Forgiveness, particularly as it applies to other human beings, is an act that makes one feel good about oneself. Positive feelings about oneself are essential to maximizing the prolife potential of others. The importance of making people feel good about themselves must never be underestimated. No matter in what stage of life we encounter man, when we positively contribute to his sense of self, we are touching the lives of countless others, some perhaps yet to be born.

REFERENCES

1. Selye, H.: The stress syndrome, American Journal of Nursing **65**:97-99, 1965.
2. Rank, O.: The trauma of birth. In Talbot, T., editor: The world of the child, Garden City, N.Y. 1968, Doubleday & Co., Inc., p. 75.
3. Tillich, P.: The courage to be, New Haven, Conn., 1952, Yale University Press, p. 44.
4. Neylan, M.: Anxiety, American Journal of Nursing **62**:110-111, 1962.
5. Brussel, J., and Irwin, T.: Depression, New York, 1973, Hawthorn Books, Inc., p. 57.
6. Branden, N.: The psychology of self-esteem, Los Angeles, 1969, Nash Publishing Corporation, p. 148.
7. Govoni, L., and Hayes, J.: Drugs and nursing implications, New York, 1965, Appleton-Century-Crofts, p. 130.
8. Branden, op. cit., p. 102.
9. Kicey, C.: Catecholamines and depressions: a physiological theory of depression, American Journal of Nursing **74**:2018-2020, 1974.

10. Yaskin, J.: Nervous symptoms as earliest manifestations of carcinoma of the pancreas, Journal of the American Medical Association **96**:1644, 1931.
11. Rice, D.: Somatic syndromes cloaking depressive states, Practitioner **183**:49, 1959.
12. Storrow, H.: The diagnosis of depression; recognizing the depressed patient. In Enelow, A., editor: Monographs of depression in medical practice, West Point, Pa., 1970, Merck Sharp & Dohme, p. 21.
13. Schwab, J.: Depression in medical and surgical patients. In Enelow, A., editor: Monographs of depression in medical practice, 1970, Merck Sharp & Dohme, p. 112.
14. Storrow, op. cit., p. 27.
15. Brussel and Irvin, op. cit., p. 61.
16. Ostow, M.: The psychology of melancholia, New York, 1970, Harper & Row, Publishers, p. 41.
17. Crary, W., and Crary, G.: Depression, American Journal of Nursing **73**:472-475, 1973.
18. Fallon, B.: And certain thoughts go through my head, American Journal of Nursing **72**:1259, 1972.
19. Bahra, R.: The potential for suicide, American Journal of Nursing **75**:1784, 1975.
20. Schneidman, E.: Preventing suicide, American Journal of Nursing **65**:111-116, 1965.
21. Litman, R.: Evaluation and management of the suicidal patient. In Enelow, A., editor: Monographs of depression in medical practice, West Point, Pa., 1970, Merck Sharp & Dohme, p. 142.
22. Durkheim, E.: Suicide: a study in sociology, New York, 1951, The Free Press, p. 14.
23. Vohen, K., and Watson, C.: Suicide in relation to time of day and days of week, American Journal of Nursing **75**:263, 1975.
24. Klugman, D., Litman, R., and Wold, C.: Suicide: answering a cry for help, Social Casework **10**:45, 1965.
25. Erikson, E.: The problem of ego identity, Journal of The American Psychoanalytic Association **4**:56-121, 1956.
26. Sullivan, H.: Infancy: the role of anxiety in the beginning differentiation of experience. In Talbot, T., editor: The world of the child, New York, 1967, Doubleday & Co., Inc., p. 96.
27. Spitz, R.: Anaclitic depression, Psychoanalytic Study of the Child **2**:313-342, 1946.
28. Williams, R., and Prugh, D.: School phobia. In Green, M., and Haggerty, R., editors: Ambulatory pediactrics, Philadelphia, 1968, W. B. Saunders Co., p. 801.
29. Brussel and Irwin, op. cit. p. 142.
30. Coleman, J., and Broen, W.: Abnormal psychology and modern life, Glenview, Ill., 1972, Scott, Foresman & Co., p. 155.
31. Toolan, J.: Suicide in children. In Green, M., and Haggerty, R., editors: Ambulatory pediatrics, Philadelphia, 1968, W. B. Saunders Co., p. 786.
32. Teicher, J.: The enigma of depression in infancy, childhood, and adolescence. In Enelow, A., editor: Monographs of depression in medical practice, West Point, Pa., 1970, Merck Sharp & Dohme, p. 47.
33. Ibid., p. 53.
34. Ibid, p. 63.
35. Mead, B.: Reactive depression in young adults. In Enelow, A., editor: Monographs of depression in medical practice, 1970, Merck Sharp & Dohme, p. 74.
36. Ibid, p. 72.
37. Coleman and Broen, op. cit., p. 348.
38. Evans, R.: Dialogue with Erik Erikson, New York, 1969, E. P. Dutton & Co., Inc., p. 53.
39. Berblinger K.: Loneliness and the depressive perspective: the chronically depressed patient. In Enelow, A., editor: West Point, Pa., 1970, Merck Sharp & Dohme, p. 162.
40. Batchelor, I.: Management and diagnosis of suicide attempts in old age, Geriatrics **10**:291-293, 1955.

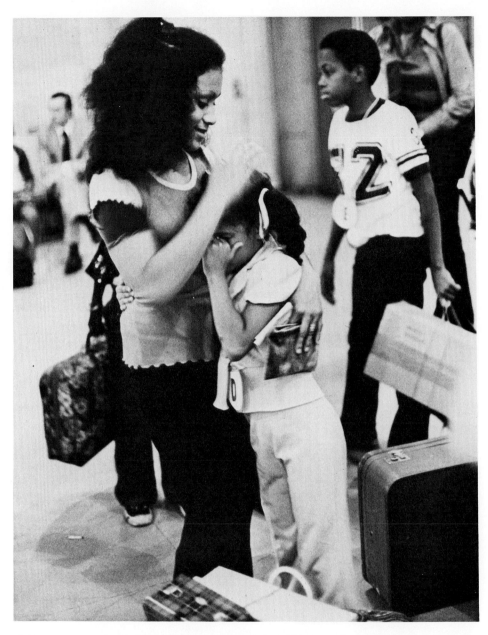

Crises are a certainty of life. The loss—or anticipated loss—of a significant relationship can create a state of disequilibrium. Adequate situational support marshals and sustains coping mechanisms and aids in resolution of the crisis and restoration of functioning to at least that of the precrisis state. Inadequate support or coping mechanisms may cause *permanent* personality disorganization. (Photograph by Dan O'Neill, Editorial Photocolor Archives.)

CHAPTER 5

Application of helping skills to selected crises

Rooted squarely in the human equation is a high ratio of stressful events that threaten emotional equilibrium. Social phenomena such as the energy and gas crises and whole cities in fiscal crisis have made the word a synonym for potential disaster. Additionally the nurse may be confronted with such medical crises as the fever crisis of penumonia and sickle-cell crisis. Change may be a major stressor! Consider some of the unexpected and sudden changes in one's life situation due to accidents, infidelity, and addiction to drugs; separations due to hospitalization, relocation, adoption, and death; and economic losses, physical losses, including sexual potency and sight, and the loss of cherished independence and autonomy. To say that at any given moment large segments of the population are on the verge of, in, or emerging from a *crisis* is not an exaggeration! Obviously the term must be recycled through a barrage of images for clarification.

DEFINITION OF CRISIS

A crisis involves an interplay of two components: the hazardous or precipitating event and the person's reaction to it. Although a crisis is not necessarily a state of illness, since man is host to crises as well as microorganisms, an analogy can be made. One can postulate with confidence that syphilis is caused by the motile spirochete *Treponema pallidum.* This conclusion satisifies the dictates of scientific inquiry, in that the organism can be isolated and hence observed in every case of the disease. Yet this spirochete does not always produce the same physiologic responses, and a small percentage of exposed individuals "experience a biologic cure" without intervention.[1] Although many external stressful situations may be identified as "crisochetes," the assumption that each person exposed exhibits the same behavior is equally erroneous. Susceptibility to the "organism" is first determined by the individual's feelings about his condition. His personal view of the situa-

109

tion makes the crisochete a pathogen or renders it innocuous. He may marshall inner resources, view the situation as a challenge, and triumph unaided; in this way a certain degree of immunity would be enjoyed. The birth of an imperfect infant is often equated with the loss of an ideal, but a woman infertile for years would not necessarily be traumatized by the condition of her baby. What constitutes a crisis is highly subjective, and the connotation does not have to be negative. According to Caplan, "the essential factor influencing the occurrence of a crisis is an imbalance between the difficulty and the importance of the problem, and the resources immediately available to deal with it."[2]

Parad and Caplan[3] define *crisis* as an acute, temporary emotional reaction to an external hazardous situation with the possible consequence of disorganizing behavior. Typically the individual in the hazardous situation responds with his traditional repertoire of coping mechanisms. Should he fail to resolve the problem rather quickly by his habitual ways of responding, the ensuing ego distress is manifested in such unpleasant emotions as uncertainty, tension, anxiety, guilt, or depression. As these unpleasant sensations mount, he turns to other resources.

If these also fail, the unrelieved emotional disequilibrium can consolidate into a severe personality disorder affecting the individual and others in the social sphere. In the simplest of terms the crisis concept may be summarized as the event (A) plus the coping resources (B) plus the meaning of the event (C) equal *crisis*![4] Crisochetes abound, and the population most at risk should be identified to help them problem solve more efficiently and avoid debilitating emotional reactions.

Distinguishing between a crisis and noncrisis is of no small import. Intervention requires that the nurse enter directly into the person's life situation. Entering into another's life space before the need to do so is validated is akin to treating a nonexistent condition. The treatment itself may well germinate complications.

Crisis intervention has a unique cluster of characteristics. A crisis brings an individual to a crossroads—a critical juncture in life. Because the internal equilibrium is off balance, he has lost his sense of direction. A crisis holds both danger and opportunity. There is peril if the hazardous situation or precipitating stress is not alleviated and the patient becomes welded to a framework of habits. Old solutions to new problems may lead to a lower level of functioning than before and to poorer mental health. Conversely, there is opportunity for emotional growth if the person in crisis is stimulated to provide novel solutions, use customary adaptive techniques in innovative fashions, and master different coping competencies. These strengths will enable better management of future stresses, as well as those problems activated by the current situation.

This, in turn, may lead to a higher level of functioning and of self-realization than existed prior to the crisis.

Many human experiences can engender great emotional turmoil; the subsequent disequilibrium *may* result in the belief that one does not have the ability to cope. Should a person newly enriched by winning a lottery find his inner resources overtaxed, his affluent state would then be one of emotional insolvency. He might deal with the situational support that he is sure to have, solicited and otherwise, by embarking on a spending spree that leaves him not only broke but also in debt to the Internal Revenue Department. Perhaps he might put distance between his social milieu and his money by buying annuities for his old age and maintaining his current job and style of life. Then again the wealth might precipitate a move to a different city and pursuit of a new career. He might purchase some underdeveloped land, play the stock markets, increase his monetary worth, start a philanthropic foundation, and run for political office.

Although crisis theory was originally formulated by mental health specialists, it is now recognized as a significant addition to the other therapeutic modalities in nursing. Meaningful intervention in a crisis situation is often predicated on a multidisciplinary approach; it is quite possible to have a nurse, social worker, and chaplain simultaneously assisting the same individual to cope with crisis. Therefore helpers must share the same frame of reference regarding techniques and objectives; to concentrate on the immediate cause of the person's disturbed equilibrium and the intervention needed to help him regain equilibrim. With no fusion of methods and goals the health providers may be left with a preponderance of data and the patient left in his dilemma.

CRISIS INTERVENTION

Life is bittersweet; crises are a part of living. Although there are nurse specialists in the art of crisis intervention, it need not be one group's special forte. In crisis intervention the nurse considers herself one resource in a group of resource persons. The first priority is recognizing an individual's petitions for assistance and then involving as many persons as possible in responding to this appeal. A nurse given the emergent task of stemming the blood flow from a gushing wound does not mistake herself for a surgeon. Yet if the nurse does not take judicious action, the surgeon's time and talent may not be needed. The expectation that nurses in general should have skill in medical emergencies and that only some nurses should have skill in emotional emergencies diametrically opposes the nursing process, which has mental health as one of its most vital humanistic components.

Notice that the time dimension of a crisis is structured. By definition, a crisis is self-limiting, lasting from 4 to 6 weeks.[5] The event that caused the crisis may have occurred from 1 to 2 weeks before help was sought or may have happened the day or night before. This recency of events mandates focusing on the presenting problem and resisting the temptation to resurrect underlying ones. Focusing on the "here and now" and helping the patient to work through his current difficulty facilitates restoration of his equilibrium to at least that of his precrisis state.

It is generally thought that during a crisis the impetus to seek relief from psychologic discomfort is maximal and defense mechanisms are less rigid. As a result, the person is more open to potential change.[6] Timely intervention and appropriate supporting services can favorably influence the outcome.

Aguilera and Messick[7] identified four steps in the process of crisis intervention that make advantageous use of the patient's motivation and readiness to resolve his problem. This reference is recommended for a more in-depth presentation. Problem solving in crisis intervention involves an assessment of the patient and his problem, planning intervention, intervention, and resolution of the crisis and anticipatory guidance. The process is a collaboration based on caring, commitment, and continuity. These ego-supportive techniques help relieve the tension, anxiety, and feelings of helplessness and hopelessness generally associated with the first impact of stress. Caring communicates a positive regard for the patient's personal definition of the experience and his feelings and potentials. Commitment is active involvement in helping the patient to manage the forces overpowering his normal homeostatic mechanisms. Because the nurse may be the one person readily accessible to the patient, she may be best able to provide continuity in a diversity of services. It would seem that, once a sense of continuity is lost, the patient becomes less motivated to disclose himself or to begin all over again. His symptoms may intensify and become more difficult to resolve than the original problem.

Assessment. Essentially the nurse is trying to understand exactly what is going on. The patient is encouraged to amplify and clarify his perception of the event, situational supports, and previous coping patterns. The nurse needs to know how the crisis has affected his life and the lives of others close to him; what actions he has already taken; to whom he turned for support and the outcome; what the similarities and differences are between this crisis and other disruptions in his life; how he usually handles disruptions; what his strengths and weaknesses are and which resources in his coping repertoire are useful and available to him now; and what his affective, or emotional, state is and how the threat to his emotional stability can be decreased in a manner compatible with his wishes, values, and aspirations. Finally, she needs to find out what the patient anticipates will happen if the obstacle to his goals persists?

Planning intervention. Utilizing data from the assessment, the patient and nurse engage in a brainstorming session to reach the short-term goal of resolving the crisis as soon as possible. A dynamic approach might be to pool their inner, interpersonal, and institutional resources, formulate and exchange hypotheses, and weigh the pros and cons of each. From this exchange of ideas the patient may see the problem in a new light and devise a constructive plan of action. The available resources and action options are also appraised as part of the long-term planning to prevent the recurrence of the crisis and to prepare the patient for coping with new ones. In tandem with this phase is helping the patient to recall how he coped with past stressful situations and to feel that his is worthy and able to plan and manage his life.

Intervention. The patient's need for help is urgently in the present, and intervention is action oriented. "Let's roll up our sleeves and see what can be done in the time we have together" is both a promise and a form of help. Brief and specific tension-reducing activities are engaged in. An especially important activity is communication that facilitates the acknowledgement, expression, and management of feelings. A joint exploration of the stressful event and its consequences is one kind of emotional catharsis that facilitates the restoration of equilibrium. Liaisons with those whom he trusts are strengthened and appropriate referrals instituted to enlarge his social system of support. The initial contact is vital, and a little help at this time is more valuable than a great deal later on. Mastery over even a minor aspect of the problem may provide the confidence and support needed to continue the struggle to make life seem whole and coherent.

Resolution of the crisis and anticipatory planning. The ego-adaptive maneuvers that proved most effective in alleviating the person's emotional discomfort are reinforced, progress made is summarized, and assistance is given in identifying other sources of support that the patient can turn to once professional help is terminated. Mutual dialogue concerning use of this experience to manage future hazardous situations is one of the most significant variables in preventive mental health. The number of planned patient-nurse contacts depends on the degree of disorganizing emotional pain, circumstances, and whether the situation endangers the life of the individual or others. In some instances and settings, one session coupled and coordinated with medical or environmental types of intervention may be sufficient to reduce emotional trauma and prevent maladaptive behavior.

Summary. Cognizance of crisis intervention techniques is not a credential for psychotherapy. Rather nurses are encouraged to master time-honored skills in problem solving and to use these skills with confidence and precision. In addition, the nurse should not be seduced by the implications that minimal effort produces maximal benefits. The highest skill is needed when on short notice the nurse is turned to for help by emotionally troubled individuals or families. There can be tremendous satisfaction in promoting life-sustaining and life-enhancing efforts of individuals by incorporating this approach to comprehensive care into other helping practices.

HELPING THE BEREAVED

Rapid, significant change or the threat of change can test contemporary man's psychic and social values to the utmost. Predictably change has been identified as the classic "precipitating event for the generation of a crisis."[8] Closely allied with change is the loss of something central to the concept of self. Loss can plunge an individual into a psychologic abyss and create a crisis of sorrow. The depth and scope of the emotional void is contingent on the degree of life disruption. Not surprisingly, the loss of mobility, vision, or other major changes in one's self-image and pattern of life can reverberate into acute mourning.

More typical of raw distress is the termination of a stable human relationship by death, especially if the terminated relationship was an essential source of need fulfillment and the deceased was relied on in innumerable ways for feelings of well-being and effective functioning.[9] The loss of a child may be more distressing than the death of an elderly or incurably ill person. The reaction to a sudden and unexpected death may be greater than to an anticipated one. Significant persons give us a sense of ourselves; their loss is much like losing a part of oneself. Great passions of love or enmity are precursors of grief; anyone hated with a passion will be missed. By contrast, if most intimate relationships were not a cadence of love and hate, there would be no need for the admonishment to "speak well of the dead."

The grieving process

Mourners, explained Engel, must traverse four normal and necessary stages as they move from anguish to acceptance.[10] Each stage makes a specific contribution to the recovery process, and none should be accelerated or eliminated if normal adaptation is to occur within a year or so.

Initial shock. The first news of actual or impending death leaves the survivor stunned and dazed. The ego is emergently anesthetized from the pain of assimilation by disbelief and denial. Denying behavior often deviates from social decorum and should not be condemned. At this time an unconscious chuckle may erupt, instead of the customary cry.[11] Dissimilar as mirth and misery are, grief is often indiscriminate. This phase persists for a few minutes to hours or even days and may be accompanied by such physiologic manifestations of overwhelming anxiety as rapid pulse, a feeling of tightness in the chest and throat, and shortness of breath.

Sometimes the person intellectually acknowledges the event and reacts with a "business-as-usual" approach, making arrangements and comforting others. This suppression or denial of the emotional impact may lead to the observation that he is "holding up well." However, admiration should be suspended if this facade is maintained.

Respect for other patients and the bereaved suggests that news of death be communicated in privacy and to the family as a group, so that they can console each other, consider, and concur in such decisions as that concerning an autopsy.

Developing awareness. Within minutes to hours the waning shock reaction is replaced by recognition of the reality and meaning of the loss. This is the time that the greatest degree of suffering is experienced and expressed. The distress may be volatile and behavior erratic, with flailing of the breast and soul-piercing wails. However, sorrow is rarely unsullied; it is tinged with guilt and hostility. "How could he leave me now?" is just as much rebuking as rhetorical. The emotions underlying unacceptable feelings toward the dead may be unleashed on the caretakers in the form of vitriolic accusations of malpractice and maltreatment. This angry, abusive behavior is not a personal denigration of the staff but rather a defense against self-abuse, which might result in mental decimation. Guilt is the litany of the living: "If only I had . . ." is a persecutory expression of failure. It is at this stage unresponsive to any realistic refutations, since all humans have the natural proclivity for leaving some things undone. Still, there may be a grain of truth in the following old and worn refrain:

> There is a sure way of telling
> From the amount of yelling
> The one who did the least
> For the deceased. . . .

Understanding the reasons for bereaved behavior requires that the nurse go with the grain rather than against it.

Crying is germane to this crisis and fulfills an important function in grief. However, voluntary suppression of tears may be due to stringent cultural inhibitions, shyness, or a natural reluctance to grieve publicly. A person in whom composure is a vital part of the self-concept should not be coerced to contrary behavior. Then, too, tears may not flow if the death was a lingering one and the outcome thoroughly anticipated. The survivors may have mourned as much as is humanly possible and completed their grief work in advance of the actual fact of death, which may bring feelings of relief, and the attendant guilt and shame may be exacerbated if the survivor is urged to behave hypocritically. Although individuals vary in its use, weeping is said to be one of the healthiest communications of anguish and its absence a cause for concern. The scourge of successful grief work is the fear that one's tears will not be sanctioned. American men are expected to hold their liquor, temper, and tears; feelings are for weaklings and women. However, solace is subsidized by compassionate acceptance. Both men and women need to feel that it is all right to cry and that the nurse will share and support their grief work.

Seeing may expedite believing, and the mourner's request to see the loved one should be honored. Institutionalizing death is a fairly recent custom, and the compulsion to take leave of the dead may be a coping pattern warranting humanitarian indulgence and accommodation. The survivor would not beseech the nurse if this were not imperative and indigenous to his manner of grieving.

Restitution. The third stage of grief work emphasizes clearly and un-equivocally the fact of death. The harsh reality of funeral and burial rites terminates denial in a public gathering. Although the need for support at the time of final separation is acknowledged, the lowering of the coffin allows for no ambiguity. Customs such as wakes and sitting shiva serve to facilitate the recovery process, the restoration of equilibrium, and reentry into the social world.

Resolving the loss. Death's aftermath leaves a defect in one's sense of continuity and wholeness. Thoughts and conversation dwell on the deceased, who in the process, achieves irreplaceable perfection—perfectly loved and perfectly loving. Since no one compares, no replacement is considered. Several months may pass before ambivalent memories become tolerable and are tolerated with less sadness and guilt. Then identification with the ideals and aspirations of the dead provide some impetus for living. Frequently identification with others who are disconsolate forms the basis for new relationships. The concern for others eventually extends to interactions disassociated with grief and to gradual replacement of the lost relationship. Emancipation from mourning is said to occur when one "remembers comfortably and realistically both the pleasures and disappointments of the relationship."[12]

Nursing implications

Understanding the normal chain of events in the grieving process helps the nurse to discern which ones are strong and supportive and which weak and in need of shoring up or missing and potentially disastrous. From such knowledge, inferences can be drawn that may be applicable to many health care settings.

Mourning can emerge whenever individuals feel their net worth depreciated. In grief work, all feelings are said to be legitimate, and their expression in human actions have wide latitude. Since the patient's diagnosis may not document a recent change, the correlation between behavior and a crisis may be overlooked; yet grieving behavior would certainly be in collusion with his other symptoms and subvert the effectiveness of prescribed therapies. Misunderstood actions are more likely to be censured. If the bereft censor their feelings as a result of their censured behavior, the repressed reality will erupt later in a mutant form. On the other hand, a rather brief inquiry may elicit feelings of sorrow and a recent loss. Supporting the person where he is in the grieving process may give him the needed stamina to struggle and search for meaningful adaptations.

Grief tugs at the heart and may threaten the nurse's own sense of equilibrium, making her feel helpless and inadequate to the task. An awkward presence is expected and preferable to composure and expertise that inures one to suffering. A central premise of crisis intervention is reliance on a variety of resources. Appropriate provision for religious rites and spiritual guidance, at times, may be the most thoughtful intervention. Thoughtful intervention also requires that we have the humility to recognize our limitations and the honesty to admit that we do not have all the answers. Bereaved family members sometimes seem impelled to conduct a disconcerting emotional inquest not relating to the medical aspects of care but rather to some indication that the staff cared about what happened—that essential strangers recognized and appreciated the worth of the deceased. Grief elicits lapses of silence, which, although there is a paucity of words, may eloquently convey all that the nurse needs to say. Sensitivity and sympathetic listening are the double helix of helping. Although hardly enough, they are always a prerequisite and bring the reverence appropriate to therapeutic communication in times of sorrow.

HELPING THE DYING
Overview

Sorrow is the legacy of living and dying; yet what we know of sorrow from personal losses and sharing the losses of others may be insufficient to help us imagine the grief that surges when one is faced with the total loss of self. Nothingness is the most difficult concept to comprehend. We cannot foresee a world without our presence, and the inconceivable is not readily coped with.

Death is un-American, and we have no dialogue for it. Americans do not die but wither and fade like a flower, pass on, or rest in peace. The buying of death insurance as life insurance epitomizes our avoidance of reality. Conditions that threaten mortality are warred on, marched against, and attacked. Death is an enemy, and these approaches hold latent promises that we shall overcome death from known and natural causes. We are lulled by the scientist's compromise with death, holding it at bay with transplants and respirators and suspending it cryogenically with techniques of "freeze-wait-reanimate."[13] A confrontation with death is catastrophic; we are caught unaware, and this victimization is associated with the crisis of all crises.

There is no comradeship between the ego and the concept of extinction. Such a repugnant idea is to be repelled—disavowed rather than endured. Man should not be expected to concede with good grace. Consequently, "all people, no matter what age they may be, automatically deal with these dreaded and dreadful emotions by *denial* ."[14]

Denial is individualized; the intellectual age, personality, and life experience determine its form and force. Having a different conceptualization of death than others, the young child reacts differently to its threat. Visual observation is part of the preschooler's work. The senses report that a buzzing fly can be muted and stilled if sprayed or swatted, but the reappearance of a look-alike fly convinces him that death is temporary and reversible. As he grows, this concept is symbolically reinforced in stories and games. True, Jack fell down and broke his crown, but up he got and home did trot. The cowboy felled by a six-shooter does not stay dead either but is resurrected in the next instant to continue the game if he wishes. In his world every relationship is "assured of being restored."[15] His sister goes off to school and returns, and his divorced father visits or can be summoned by phone. The same baby-sitter comes each morning when his mother leaves for work and departs only when his mother returns. There is constancy and predictability in absences, and separations are only for the time being, which is fairly short and definite.

In the world of the child, there are no chance occurrences; children cause things to happen. Fairy tales and cartoons amuse and admonish; they reinforce beliefs that children are punished for misdeeds by banishment or abandonment and that death in the form of a person may swoop down on them and threaten mutilation. This person may be a boogeyman, a monstrous gorilla, an ogre, or the devil. Death is also a god, whose whereabouts and first name no one seems to know. This god sends angels down for people at will. Catapulted from home to hospital, the child thinks that he is being abandoned; pain and immobility are additional reprisals for misdeeds. Some of this anxiety may be worked through in fantasy, since in fairy tales deliverance always occurs.

In the young child's mind he and his loved ones function as a unit, and his response to separation is total and absolute. The time between visits seem interminable, and he wonders why those he depends on for care and comfort allow strangers to hurt him. Although he has no real awareness of personal death, the anxiety engendered by the separation is similar to death anxiety. One means of tolerating the distress is the repression of all feelings for the loved ones, and the child may barely notice when they visit or when they leave. Denial of separation is symbolically denial of death, and the child may become a familiar figure of bereavement.

Even when the tensions and anxieties are eased by constant parental attendance, the dying child responds to their anguish and fears; "his parent's feelings become his feelings."[16] When his parents are sad and depressed, he is sad and depressed. Because he must bear some of the agony communicated to him by others, in addition to the discomforts of his illness, the task of dying may become burdensome, although its impersonality and permanence are not yet realized.

When the child begins to comprehend that death is final and irreversible is a moot question. Seemingly when a maturing child grasps even faintly the reality of existence as a unique individual, he cannot avoid the question of where he came from and where he must go. Sometimes the child is 4, 5, or 6 years of age before he has a stable concept of self, and at this stage the concept of identity arouses disturbing feelings about the possible loss of identity. At this time he can be deeply upset by an illness that threatens existence, and much emotional strength is used to deny the relentless reality of a final separation. When denial is no longer completely effective, disturbance is shown by restlessness and uncontrolled, angry outbursts; and his death is often "heralded by increasingly unsettled behavior."[17] It is thought that from 5 to 10 years of age, children begin to accommodate themselves to the propositon that personal death can be a irrevocable solution to some accidents and illnesses, and by the age of 10 the adult concept is fairly well established. On first realizing that the integrity and intactness of the body cannot be regained, the child "passes through identical stages of dying as the adult whether or not the knowledge is explicitly conveyed or gradually deduced."[18]

Stages of grieving behavior

Denial is the adult's version of magical thinking and includes the young child's belief of causation; not facing sad facts will cause the odds against one to be reduced. In addition to denial, awareness that life is imminently finite may evoke four other manifestations of grief: anger, bargaining, depression, and finally acceptance.[19] Being full of paradoxes, man tends to complicate any systematized ordering of events; thus the stages may overlap and sometimes go back and forth.

Moreover, the process of becoming aware may also be a series of sequential steps; progressing from closed awareness to suspicious awareness, mutual pretense, and open awareness.[20] *Closed awareness* is the most likely reaction at the beginning of a fatal illness. Even though others may know, the person has no inkling of the true nature of his condition and continues to plan optimistically for the future. However, the suspicion that life may be in jeopardy is soon aroused by such cues as increasing pain and weakness, transfer to a special setting for special therapy, and evasive answers to questions. Having made some determinations of the seriousness of his illness, *suspicious awareness* may progress to that of *mutual pretense*, or the patient may begin to grieve in fearful aloneness.

The stance of mutual pretense is adopted when the patient and staff tacitly agree to refrain from any discussion of the patient's true condition. Mutual pretense can be advantageous to the patient.[21] Refusing to share the realization of fatal illness makes the thought less real or potent. By not conversing about impending death, the patient can push the idea into the back of his mind, where it excites fewer anxieties. This pretense may be his way of sparing himself the emotional agony of verbalizing his fate and making his dying as comfortable as possible for him. In the privacy of his mind the patient may be honest with himself but instinctively sense that precise information concerning his fatal diagnosis and prognosis may diminish his personal hopes. Subsequent therapeutic efforts would be meaningless because in a sense they would be directed toward a hopeless cause. Furthermore, the patient may trust and feel more secure with a nurse who is sensitive enough to understand and meet his needs without disregarding his preference for keeping his knowing unconfirmed.

Should either the nurse or the patient decide to end the pretense, the situation would become one of *open awareness,* in which the shock and disbelief of *"no, not me!"* becomes an acknowledged *"yes, me"* between the patient and the nurse. To facilitate this acknowledgment, some believe that the patient should be encouraged to give up his denial, described as a state of isolation in which his concerns may be heightened. The crux of this phase is the value judgment that an individual apprised of the seriousness of his illness and its probable outcome is more likely to die a peaceful and dignified death; the patient is given the opportunity to make appropriate plans and decisions and to set his house in order. The disclosure can be made with hope—that something can be done about his problem and to relieve his suffering. The words *dying* and *death* do not have to be mentioned at all.

"To tell or not to tell" should not dichotomize nursing intervention. It is not even the question, since a question's appropriateness is dependent on the person to whom it is addressed. A more meaningful inquiry is how to create a patient-nurse relationship that allows the patient to open up topics heretofore deemed improper and to "announce his dying if he chooses."[22] This kind of interaction is more likely to occur if the patient senses that the nurse will help him to cope with emerging feelings of such personal magnitude. Helping the patient cope may involve more listening than talking. Listening is always at the patient's convenience. To think that the patient can dwell on his impending death 24 hours a day is illogical; he may often revert to denial to help him maintain the slender hold on his values, self-image, and self-esteem. Then, too, he is selective in communicating his distress and least likely to drop his defenses in front of individuals whose distress and denial match his own.

The awareness of *"yes, me"* may cause him to rage at man and God: of all the people in the world *"why me?"* Why must he be the one to relinquish his dreams and aspirations and the companionship of family and friends? The list of grievances is long and his indignation great because no argument can rationally answer his questions. The rage from his sense of impotence seeks dissipation and when outwardly projected on others is likely to provoke the least helpful response of rejection. Hostile demands evoke further remonstrances and dissatisfaction. Efforts to make him comfortable are construed as deliberate efforts to sabotage his well-being. Nothing pleases: the bed is too high, too low, or too flat and the room too hot, too cold, or too warm. It is especially difficult to encourage the ventilation of anger when one may well be the target, but this is the approach that would be most helpful. Acrimony is a normal rebuttal to death. Understanding the course and the cause of the patient's anger may better help the nurse to subordinate her own. Once the angry thoughts lose some of their force, the patient will make fewer unreasonable demands on the nurse, but his grief will assume a less noticeable form. *"Yes, me, but*—if you do this for me, I will do that for you" ushers in the third stage of bargaining. This is a relatively private period of negotiating, sometimes with the staff but more often with God in hopes of postponing the inevitable. Maybe God, who ignored the angry supplications, will be more favorably disposed if approached nicely. From childhood one has learned that good behavior sometimes leads to the granting of a special wish. Thus "I promise not to miss a Sunday attending Mass from now on" perhaps, just perhaps, may lead to an extension of life.

When the patient becomes sequestered in silence, the *"yes, me, but . . ."* has been denuded to *"yes, me."* This awareness culminates in a deep and sorrowful depression. Convulsed with sadness, the patient may be found sobbing or with tears streaming down his face. As he slowly prepares himself for the loss of everything, he talks less and is less able to interact with a variety of people. A presence that comfortably supports him in silence may enhance his emotional preparation for what lies ahead. In this fourth stage, pain may be one of the certainties.[23] The psychic pain of depression may be displaced to the idea of bodily pain and potentiate the preexisting organic pain. On the other hand, organic pain may intensify a depressive reaction by reminding the patient of his helplessness in staying the threat to his life. When it becomes obvious that treatment has been unsuccessful in halting the disease, complaints of intractable pain can be an assurance of securing help in a euphemistic fashion without articulating the now predominant fears of loneliness and abandonment. Thus, by making known her availability in a continuing relationship, the nurse can provide a great deal of comfort in the face of uncertainty. Pain is impure and seldom presents itself or can be treated alone.

Patients usually do not overrate their pain and should have an essential say in its management long before they are overwhelmed or exhausted by the disease process. Individualized care means that the patient chooses those periods when he desires to be alert and have maximal control over his environment and when he prefers drug-induced tranquility and somnolence. The anticipation of pain intensifies it. If pain is kept in constant remission, the patient is less likely to develop a tolerance to drugs. Since pain itself is the strongest antagonist to analgesia, its intrusion warrants more vigorous treatment. The stress of pain can increase the production of epinephrine and lead to such untoward physiologic responses as increased heart rate and cardiac output.[24] Prolonged pain reduces the capacity to maintain homeostasis; the latter is maintained as long as conditions support a constant internal environment. The patient who needs a potent analgesic should not be deprived of relief because of the nurse's overconcern with the possibility of drug addiction. Few, if any, medical regimens pose no risk. More credible may be ethical concern with side effects of narcotics, such as respiratory depression to which the patient may eventually succumb. On the other hand, we tend to dismiss with a supreme air of forgetfulness the dangerous drugs dispensed to treat the disease, although such chemicals not only threaten life but also impair the quality of that remaining.

Sufficient time and help in working through the previous phases of grieving may prepare the patient to "contemplate his coming end with a certain degree of quiet expectation."[25] Acceptance is almost devoid of feelings; the individual is neither happy nor terribly sad, angry nor depressed. There is little pain or discomfort, and, as in life's beginning, there is a great need for sleep. Yet, neither fearing nor despairing, "even the most accepting, the most realistic patients left the possibility open for some cure, for the discovery of a new drug" or sudden success in a research project.[26]

Seemingly, then, *strong* hopes do not inspire the type of problem solving that leads to acceptance. If the individual's habitual way of coping was to meet a problem head-on, he may enlarge on this method of adaptation and engage in a splendid struggle for survival. Although his dying may not conform to a preferred proposition, who is to criticize the path he takes to keep his appointment in Samarra? Must we insist on our preconceptions or is "the struggle not to die as much a successful adjustment for some" as acceptance is for others?[27]

The patient should not be exhorted to resolve personal conflicts between himself and others or set his house in order according to our values either. He should be allowed to assume any reasonable role that he chooses as long as his mental faculties are not clouded by drugs, anesthesia, or disease. The patient confers whatever rights and privileges the family and staff have in his bedside arena. Truly loving family relationships do emerge at the time of death often enough to be considered a norm. However, in a conflict between needs of the family and those of the patient, the latter's have priority. This is not a callous attitude but, if nothing else, a realistic concession to time.

Life can be described as a continuum: a finite linear measurement with a prologue and an epilogue. It commences with birth and continues as one grows, matures, ages, and dies. It is a sequential process with a beginning and an end. Consider, however, two basic physical entities: matter and energy. All the activities of matter are the result of energy changes. Examples of energy transactions abound, with the electrocardiogram and the electroencephalogram being but two. Matter, then, can be reduced to energy, *but* energy cannot be destroyed—only transformed. Thus there is another way to describe life. Rather than thinking of it in terms of a straight line leading to extinction, one may also view it as curvilinear with a merging of energy—that of

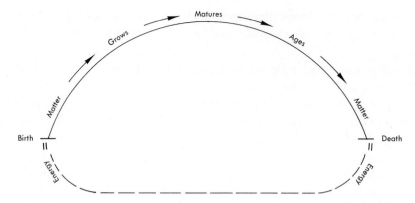

Life cycle: a continuum. (Courtesy Professor Joyce A. Ellis, R.N., M.S., Purdue University School of Nursing, Lafayette, Ind.)

the end with the beginning—closure and infinity. (See accompanying illustration.)

REFERENCES

1. Holvey, D., and Talbott, J.: The Merck manual of diagnosis and therapy, West Point, Pa., 1972, Merck Sharp & Dohme, p. 1537.
2. Caplan, G.: Principles of preventive psychiatry, New York, 1964, Basic Books, Inc., Publishers, p. 39.
3. Parad, H., and Caplan, G.: A framework for studying families in crisis. In Parad, H., editor: Crisis intervention: selected readings, New York, 1965, Family Service Association of America, p. 66.
4. Hill, H.: Generic features of families under stress. In Parad, H., editor: Crisis intervention: selected readings, New York, 1965, Family Service Association of America, p. 40.
5. Aguilera, D., and Messick, J.: Crisis intervention: theory and methodology, St. Louis, 1974, The C. V. Mosby Co., p. 16.
6. Oberst, M.: The crisis-prone staff nurse, American Journal of Nursing 75:1920, 1973.
7. Aguilera and Messick, op. cit., p. 57.
8. Hall, J., and Weaver, B.: Crisis: a conceptual approach to family nursing, In Hall, J., and Weaver, B., editors: Nurs-ing of families in crisis, Philadelphia, 1974, J. B. Lippincott Co., p. 4.
9. Engel, G.: Grief and grieving; the dying patient: a nursing perspective, New York, 1972, The American Journal of Nursing Co., p. 107.
10. Ibid., pp. 108-110.
11. Epstein, C.: Nursing the dying patient, Reston, Va. 1975, Reston Publishing Co., p. 64.
12. Engel, op. cit., p. 112.
13. Cutler, F.: Coming to terms with death, Chicago, 1974, Nelson-Hall Co., p.32.
14. Easson, W.: The dying child, Springfield, Ill., 1972, Charles C Thomas, Publisher, p. 10.
15. Kavanaugh, R.: Facing death, Los Angeles, 1972, Nash Publishing Corporation, p. 129.
16. Easson, op. cit., p. 24.
17. Ibid., p. 12.
18. Kavanaugh, op. cit., p. 139.
19. Kübler Ross E.: What is it like to be dying? American Journal of Nursing 71:54-61, 1971.
20. Glasser, B., and Strauss, A.: Awareness contexts and social interaction, American Sociological Review 29:669-679, 1964.

21. Verwoerdt, A., and Wilson, R.: Communication with fatally ill patients: Tacit or explicit? American Journal of Nursing **67**:2307-2309, 1967.
22. Kavanaugh, op. cit., p. 67.
23. Woodforde, J., and Fielding, J.: Pain and cancer. In Weisenberg, M., editor: Pain: clinical and experimental perspectives, St. Louis, 1975, The C. V. Mosby Co., p. 330.
24. Copp, L.: The spectrum of suffering, American Journal of Nursing **74**:491-495, 1974.
25. Kübler-Ross, E.: On death and dying, New York, 1969, Macmillan Publishing Co., Inc., p. 99.
26. Ibid., p. 123.
27. Sharp, D.: Lessons from a dying patient, American Journal of Nursing **68**:1517-1520, 1968.

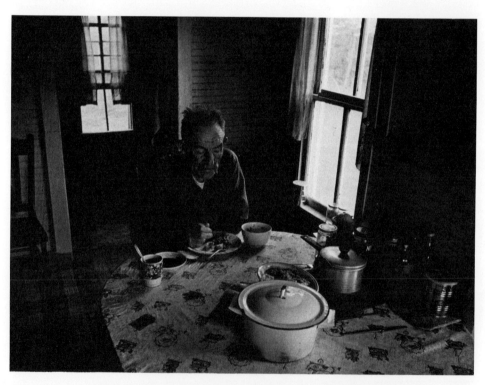

Life can be lonely. Deviations from the norms of youth and physical perfection may cause individuals to be discredited and devalued—isolated as imperfect facsimiles of other human beings. When the sender and receiver of messages are one and the same, life may stagnate—no discoveries or renewals. Loneliness is the tyranny of a clock—intoning time that cannot be filled. (Photograph by Michael Smith, Editorial Photocolor Archives.)

CHAPTER 6

Common crises in the presentation of self

To the blind, "loss of sight is a dying!"[1] The deaf are bewildered by their feelings of "deadness."[2] The individual with kidney failure often "feels he might as well be dead" rather than live a life dependent on chronic dialysis.[3] The loss of a body part or function is an assault on the body-mind-spirit, pure and whole, and often a requiem to a way of life that was one with the person. Man cannot separate these kinds of losses from feelings of some loss of self because many areas of former self-sufficiency are irrevocably altered.

He is now one of the handicapped—stigmatized and discredited as deformed, maimed, or crippled. Whatever delicate balance was achieved between himself and society has been torn asunder, and the latter offers little to cushion his shock except the company of others who share his ordeal. The self that the individual now presents may be a social pariah because handicapped people arouse in the unafflicted vague feelings of anxiety.[4] We cannot escape it. The knowledge and fear vibrate within us that, but for capricious chance, such could be our lot. We can deny and rationalize it beyond recognition, but handicapped people constantly remind us of our own vulnerability. To repudiate this unbidden identification we tend to banish the disabled to the margins of our attention. Therefore not only must the handicapped individual adjust to body changes and a new way of feeling about himself but also with patience and pain must learn to adjust to social attitudes toward him.

BODY IMAGE: ITS IMPORTANCE AND IMPLICATIONS

Man is a mélange of psychologic, physiologic, and sociologic experiences that cohere into a mental self-representation. This self-image is a condensed formulation, or summary, of a whole range of beliefs, attitudes, ideals, and expectancies concerning life and life roles. In the concept of "I" and self, body image, or somatic ego, is an integral part of identity. Body image is the dynamic interaction of genetic endowments "with the many experiences the individual has in the process of defining his identity."[5] Body imagery may be a more appropriate construct to describe the unconscious mental representation and belief system that one has about the structure and sensations of one's body and the significance of the parts of the body in evaluating space and moving about freely in the environment. Like other self-perceptions molded by social interaction, man's model of himself may be accurate or inaccurate and favored or faulted.

There are norms concerning the appearance and management of one's body, and individuals see themselves in terms of this cultural mirror. Body image also may be considered three-dimensional, encompassing the ideal, public, and real image of the individual. Although conceptually simplified, body image has many subtle and complex manifestations. One complexity to remember is that the concept that one forms of one's body is often converted into a conviction.

An idealized body image includes all the values and attitudes that a person has acquired with respect to what his body ought to be—how he thinks he should appear, sound, smell, and function. In the United States the emphasis is on youth, vitality, physique, wholeness, and constant activity.[6] We spell out with excruciating candor the desirable functions and measurements of the human form, and with the same calipers we tend to judge character. Not surprisingly we have become virtual Picassos in the art of presenting in prominent relief a public image of desirability and acceptability. Using "identity kits" of cosmetics, clothing, and colognes, we try to exude auras, if not evidence, of our personal merits. In pursuit of a contour we bribe our bodies with vitamins and minerals to sustain our efforts to exercise and reduce.

A realistic body image must lie somewhere between narcissism and hypochondriasis. Self-love provides the motivation to potentiate strengths and improve shortcomings. Health conservation is a crucial variable in all competencies and accommodations to growth and change. A balance between self-love and good health enables one to accept one's body without undue preoccupation. Self-acceptance, conceding that the ideal body image may not be achievable, frees a person to cultivate and nurture all his marvelously authentic human assets.

An intriguing aspect of body imagery is the view the individual holds of his exterior and interior. The exterior is the most distinguishable demarcation between the self and others and the first line of defense against the impact of unwanted stimuli. Psychologically a person is more aware of his exterior and can visualize it and control its musculature.

A break in the body surface, whether caused by accident or intentional surgery, is a loss of continuity and a threat to safety. By contrast, the body's interior is perceived as being less specialized for dealing with the immediate environment and to a large extent is a somewhat mysterious realm of involuntary responses.

Tangible evidence that the striated musculature of the exterior can be made rigid to prevent penetration is available to any nurse who gives an injection, but the degree to which individuals can manipulate muscles to contain emotions may be less well known. Arthritic patients have been noted to express "hostility" rarely and "even in situations of considerable frustration" to maintain their "affability."[7] Some of their symptoms may derive from efforts to prevent the outbreak of volatile emotions that may be catastrophic to their self-image. By converting their exterior into resistant retaining walls, they restrain disturbing impulses and feelings.

Loss of a body part or function

An important consideration applicable to body image is the difference between a congenital defect and one acquired in adolescence or later.[8] A congenital or early handicap may be incorporated into the self-concept as a *lack*, instead of a *loss*, during the process of growth and development. These handicaps do not seem to have the same emotional connotations as do disabilities sustained in later life; the very young are less likely to suffer the comparison between present body image and a previous one. The school nurse might anticipate that well-meaning suggestions to correct "crossed eyes, buck teeth, and pigeon toes" may be resisted if such body changes are too threatening to the highly valued "me."

Socially the masculine image is still associated with production, and despite the rebellion against some of the stifling aspects of the role, the feminine image relates more explicitly to reproduction. Although a male should be a blend of character and charisma, face and figure are said to be the female's fortune. Feminine self-essence has so thoroughly incorporated the uterus and the breast that their removal is seen as mutilation.[9] Although individuals respond in unique ways to the same operation, generally the excision of these organs represents to them some loss of femininity and sexuality. The postmastectomy breast prosthesis helps the patient to maintain privacy concerning the disfigurement and prevents her relegation to a devalued group.

Facial disfigurements, such as those caused by radical head and neck surgery or severe burns, are the most highly visible of all body changes and are devastating to body image. In addition to other concerns, the individual whose looks have been radically altered is extremely sensitive to the reactions of others to the change and the impact of the disability on face-to-face communication. Paradoxically, because the disability is evident to everyone, the person may more readily accept it.[10] Concealment maneuvers, which increase intrapersonal stress, are unnecessary, and this reduction in such stress may minimize some of the tension in social interactions. Moreover, what is obviously discernible may be more frankly discussed, and some of the highly charged emotions concerning the disfigurement are dissipated.

Americans place a high value on mobility. An infant's first step brings pride and praise. A great emotional investment is made in those parts of the body related to this function. Consider the phantom limb phenomenon. After the loss of a limb, some patients continue to complain of pain in that part.[11] The source of the pain has been variously attributed to irritation of nerve endings by scar tissue or neural excitation from dilating and constricting blood vessels. Now, however, this is thought possibly to be an example of the person's central body image dramatically failing to corroborate the loss of one of its parts and denying it by distorting the meaning of stimuli. Once a person has passed through the difficult process of socialization, the central body image is well formed, and any organ can be retained in fantasy. Phantom sensations may occur in other body parts that are surgically or accidentally removed. The experience is frightening because rationally the patient knows that the part no longer exists. Body misperceptions of arms and legs may be more openly acknowledged than are misperceptions of breasts and reproductive organs. Patients seem reluctant and ashamed to focus further attention on these private parts of their anatomy.

Just as amputations cause changes in body configuration, such conditions as emphysema may also impair dexterity in movement. Invisible losses may cause less interpersonal tension if the symptoms can be managed unobtrusively. The cough of emphysema or the sight of sputum communicates negative information; the person would need to persuade those around him that the condition is not contagious. An abrupt loss is said to be more traumatic than a gradual one—for example, crippling accidents as opposed to crippling arthritis. Gradual losses may allow more time for adjusting to the effects of altered activity levels and body image. However, this depends on the extent to which one's life is disrupted. Spinal cord injuries resulting in paralysis cause major problems in adjustment and adaptation. Disabilities, such as multiple sclerosis, that are characterized by periods of exacerbation and remission are difficult to accept and interpret. Any change in symptoms may convince a patient that he is on the way to total disability or recovery. The adjustment to a gradual loss is often impeded by false kindness in the attempt to spare the patient grief; yet hope is essential if he is not to resign himself to an apathetic social death. Adjustment to surgical losses begins preoperatively. Priority is given to helping the patient and others significant in his social sphere before the loss occurs to begin the rebuilding necessary to reconstruct a whole life. Body image problems are predictable in many patient-care situations; sensitivity to their occurrence may help the nurse to intervene more effectively in their prevention and resolution. The nurse's concern and interest may motivate the patient and his relatives to "rekindle and renew mutual respect for their likenesses and differences, their shared and separate needs."[12]

Congruent with a positive body image is the ability to function with control for time and place.[13] The ability to use one's body functionally to achieve exactly what was intended wins plaudits for the skilled worker, sports hero, and ballet dancer. Functional control achieved in early development becomes assimilated into the self-image and is taken for granted until lost. Beyond early childhood the control of bowel and bladder functions is not an impressive accomplishment but a habitual way of responding. Even the preoccupied first grader who accidentally wets his pants on the playground deviates from the norm. So inconsistent is this mishap with body image that he feels betrayed. Because the body houses the self, he is ashamed of himself, a shame made more merciless because this loss of control was witnessed.

How colostomies must scald the psyche! Personality disruption is bound to occur to some degree when the body's surface is disrupted by a seemingly autonomous orifice that erupts waste products with dependable irregularity. The patient often communicates that the aberrant structure does not belong to him by naming his stoma *"old stinky"* or *Mt. Vesuvius* and refusing to care for or look at it. The nurse should keep in mind that the patient may be more reasonable than recalcitrant from his point of view. Why should he learn self-care for something not a part of himself? Time is needed to reconstruct a new body image when one's central one has been shattered. Time is needed to learn the management of malodorous body secretions, to control information about the condition, and to begin the arduous process of resocialization.

Replacement of a body part

Transplantation procedures involve the introduction of a foreign organ into the patient's body. Unlike a prosthesis of visible, inanimate material, an alien heart or kidney is embedded deep inside the body beyond control and untouched except in fantasy. Tourkow[14] emphasizes a fundamental psychologic difference between traditional and transplant operations. In traditional surgery a life is saved by the *removal* of an organ, and the body image is *constricted*. In transplantation an organ is *added* to the body with the implication that life has been extended because something has been given. Thus life-extending operations necessitate the *extension* of the body image to incorporate the new organ psychologically into one's body concept.

The self is not distinct from the body but of it, and transplantation operations present new problems for the psyche. Of the many operations, including corneal and liver transplantations, the cardiac and renal seem to typify the commonalities in patient-care situations best. First, mention must be made of the difference between the candidates for these two types of surgery. Although they both may have critical organ failure, the body image of the patient with cardiac disease is radically dissimilar to that of the other. The heart is the dominant body organ—the symbol of life and love. The conscious self makes little distinction between any heart disease and extinction. Moreover, no organ failure is analogous to the "silent coronary." Therefore heart disease is the metaphor for sudden mortality. Ravaged by anxieties, the heart transplantation candidate must undergo a grave eleventh hour procedure dependent on organ retrieval from the dead. Conversely, except in rare instances the patient with kidney disease has two organs and could survive with one. Should both kidneys fail, he may have sufficient resilience to adjust to dialysis for years. Because the donor could be living, the patient's life does not inhere in another's death.

Gifts, however, imply obligations, especially those given at great human expense. Whether the donor was living or dead, the organ immediately, in the mind, represents another human being, and the recipient feels an obligation to him and his family.[14] Often he has the inner conviction that he has to become in some way like the donor. Some gifts are acknowledged with guilt; the recipient may doubt whether he is entitled to the organ. The technologic intervention that keeps deceased donor organs functioning also raises doubts concerning the definition of death. As a result the recipient may consider the donor symbolically living-dead and himself a robber. The living donor, however, can decide freely.

Gratitude may be expressed with euphoria or seeming indifference. Many transplant patients express the feeling of being reborn, and this belief almost borders on the delusional.[14] Other patients may deny that the donated organ has any emotional significance and thereby somewhat defer dealing with the paradox of simultaneously extending the body image and gaining stability.

Gifts may be refused if the donor is disliked or the recipient is a very private person who unconsciously views such gifts as intrusions. Seemingly some acute rejection responses can be attributed to "psychologic processes influencing physiologic mechanisms."[14] The emotional edicts encountered in making body changes harmonious with body concepts find parallels in substance in transplantation patients. They must mourn the loss of a necessary-to-life organ or function and cope with the fear of death and of the future. They must extend their central body image, when the body they are familiar with is debauched by drugs and disabilities—all this while they may be feeling some obligation to the person who is now a part of themselves.

But what of the living donor? Outside the surgical arena, he tends to be forgotten. In conjunction with the surgical trauma is the dual emotional trauma of losing a part of oneself and coping with fantasies concerning what happens to a part of the body when it is being used by someone else. The living donor also has to face the possibility that a valuable and irreplaceable part of him may be rejected, and, if this part malfunctions in another, he has to reconcile himself to the fact that no gain was substituted for the loss. Transplantation procedures may have severe preoperative and postoperative impact on the donor, who is frequently a family member. It is extremely difficult for a capable relative to refuse donation without feeling directly responsible for the recipient's chronic condition or death. Feelings of hostility, personal deprivation, and grief may develop before and after the procedure and be defended against by constant discussion of benefits to the recipient. If bland optimism continually masks strong, ambivalent feelings, with the donor perceiving the procedure alternately as malevolent and destructive and as life giving and enriching, the donor's sense of isolation and loneliness may intensify. His sense of stability will not admit hostility toward the recipient and misgivings about the surgery. Presenting the donor with a hypothetical transplantation situation may enable the projection and safe ventilation of strong feelings concerning the loss and fears of death or organ rejection. The nurse needs to help the donor and other relatives to recognize and accept uncomfortable feelings as normal human responses to stress.

Allow an addendum. The centrality of the concept of physical wholeness to American life may have a corollary in our reluctance even after death to donate organs, permit autopsies, and be cremated.

BODY IMAGE AND THE LONELY SELF

> So lonely, the words do not come—footsteps in the hall—
> Someone on his way to somewhere—mocking me in my room of nowhere—
> So lonely, the words have no meaning—the future is still—
> A dead world holding corpses—bearing mine among them . . .*

Monologues by the muses do not necessarily move the masses, and for many people life is a saga of sameness. When the present merges uninterruptedly with the future, sameness becomes more dreaded than solitude. Loneliness grows, and in the nature of some growths it can seriously compromise survival potential. "Loneliness for a person any age is a situation threatening to the personality." It assaults the body with fear, frustration, resentment, anger, mistrust, fatigue, colds, and ulcers.[15] The loneliness arbitrarily inflicted by social rejection may cause intractable pain. Man can surmount serious hardships as long as he has human contact and concern. Most people simply do not have sufficient emotional collateral to revise and rebuild a body image in isolation.

Loneliness is part of the human condition. A few specific conditions should suffice to illuminate the subject. The loneliness of emotional illness may be due in part to inadequacy in interpersonal relationships and to stigmatization by the public. Like other human beings the person with a mental disability wants to be accepted and understood but may be more hesitant and fearful of forming new relationships. Once recovered, however, he risks being discredited unless information concerning his disability is socially controlled. There is hardly any distinguishing characteristic about the dialogue between a former patient and another person until the disability is divulged. Such remarks as "I had no idea he was crazy; he sounded so normal" show the irrational prejudgments against mental illness. Highly sensitive and easily hurt, the formerly disabled knows that misunderstood communications are likely to be interpreted as symptoms of disease. Inability to manage the tension in interpersonal relationships may result in mutual avoidance by the patient and others. Perhaps the nurse may be most helpful by encouraging the patient to enforce his rights to privacy and mention his disability to inquisitors only when necessary or when he wishes to do so. Labels are hard to dislodge. Instead of labeling people as *confused* or *crazy,* we should regard them as human beings coping as best they know how with their life situations. Negative labels limit opportunities to develop closeness with anyone and may lead to a barren existence.

---

*From Ferguson, D.: The lonely self, American Journal of Nursing **73:**1757, 1973.

Human beings are destined to age and die. In the last stages of the life cycle the body image is under constant siege. Biologic changes, acute or insidious in onset, culminate in diminished physical abilities and powers of perception. Former bonds with work, family, friends, and neighborhood may be broken by retirement, separation, ill health, and death. When no significant substitution for loss of social support can be found, the elderly may succumb to a life of lonely social obsolescence—obsolescence because society values youthful productive citizens and devalues passive consumers. The aged, no longer able to fulfill their accustomed roles, may be institutionalized or left to live alone in circumstances of intolerance and isolation. For some older persons, disengagement, or the gradual withdrawal from social interaction, may be an expression of their personalities; more often, social changes and altered body image deteriorate the quality of human relationships and leave little alternative to aloneness. Intrinsic to the nursing process is awareness of the nurse's own attitudes toward aging and the aged and appreciation of the many ways in which their strengths, courage, and faith may be used to help them live more satisfying lives. We need to develop more skill in working with the increasing number of persons in this phase of the life cycle. We need to become active against the stigmas that segregate the elderly from the mainstream of life.

In terms of emotional devastation and interpersonal relationships, two of the most distressing disabilities may be the loss of vision and hearing. Human existence after the loss of sight and sound can become an odyssey of empty hours uncomplicated by choice, challenge, or companionship.

To see and hear are normal; people who do not are considered abnormal. The public rarely considers that individuals with these handicaps are normal persons under abnormal circumstances and that they differ from one another as do the members of a heterogeneous group.

Living is too complex; there is little time for true *involvement*. When a breach opens in the normal channels of communication, it is likely to be spanned with apologetic pity. Pity, in this instance, is only a filigree of a feeling flung in passing, although the giver may canonize it as compassion. Pity can be serenely offered, since it prevents the arousal of deep emotions and satisfies one's conscience for keeping a safe distance from the blind and deaf. Thus when faces go unseen or the world becomes incredibly quiet, the normal continuum of human relationships for the blind and deaf may be broken.

Loss of sight

The eye is "I." Conjoined, they symbolize wholeness. "Of all the messages reaching the brain, nine out of ten" are visual.[16] To become suddenly blind is to be ricocheted backward to a time when one could not sign one's name, read one's mail, tell time, dial a phone, button a sweater correctly, tell the right shoe from the left, distinguish between paper money, and feed oneself without spilling. It is to be mesmerized in immobility. Because the outer world is in constant motion, objects do not rest secure. Their shape, size, and position become indiscernible.

Life has lost its landscape. For some it is neither light nor dark, but neutral gray. Perceptions that once brought pleasure, such as familiar faces or trendy fashions, have melded into a background of monotony. Time is measureless, and the present passes by unnoticed. The days may be getting shorter and new car models may be on the street. So much information can be garnered in the normal course of coming and going. Social discourse dependent on direct observation or reading becomes difficult. In a swiftly changing social order, one who converses too much about the old is a bore, and one who knows nothing new is dull. The blind individual must relinquish cherished forms of recreation at a time when they are most needed: no more swimming, hiking, driving, playing cards, or bowling.

Economic doors are slammed: he will likely lose his job. Expenses mount: cabs, rather than public conveyances, delivery of goods, and housekeeping services may be necessities. Further eroding the self-image is the inability to intermingle freely as just another face in the crowd. Guide dogs, a white cane, and dark glasses are the optics of the outcast. People who brush up against him now pause to scrutinize him. Crowds, too, create social schisms.

Seeing is believing, a means of "making sure," or verifying the information received by our other senses. While sitting at the table, we can tell by touch the difference between a napkin and a piece of bread. However, before choosing either, we unconsciously glance to make sure. If the bread has an unfamiliar taste or smell, we automatically examine it with our eyes. Sight is the censor of our other senses. Contrary to popular belief, the loss of one sense is not automatically compensated for by the quickening of another. In reality, increased sense efficiency is due to increased effort, concentration, training, and use. The individual who has lost his sight also loses confidence in his other senses and discredits his body as having little potential for future performance. So painful are such losses that he is persuaded that life from now on must be lived posthumously.

Communication barriers. Usually, when two sighted persons meet, each has the option of making conversational overtures. Since a blind patient cannot identify other people or their exact location, he feels he can speak only when spoken to. Once engaged in conversation, he cannot validate any of the speakers' remarks by their body language. Thus, to discern the meaning of a simple remark, "Hi, you look just great," may not be so simple. Although a warm smile might make it a compliment, a sneer or smirk would make it a gross insult. Our faces mirror the nuances of most messages. Since the blind have no such mirrors, the normal give and take of facial interaction is missing. In response to the greeting, a fixed smile may be as inappropriate as a poker face; so the blind person may adopt a bland expression until he can get a better feel for the conversation. If he misinterprets the message, he knows that verbal communication has failed him.

There is yet another factor. The lack of facial feedback can be disconcerting to the sighted person, who is clueless concerning the reception of his comment. Along with minimal facial activity comes seemingly total immobility. At first the nurse may notice only that something is missing. Further observation may identify the missing element as that of gesturing. Some gestures have become so ordinary that they are scarcely noticed, but the blind patient cannot animate his conversation for fear of knocking something over. Describing an object as "this wide" may overturn his water pitcher; and he would feel foolish if he pointed while saying, "Please hand me my comb," because he cannot be certain of its position. The patient's lack of ease in the use of body language presents an enigma that makes others uneasy. Because individuals tend to fear what they do not understand, the blind person is avoided.

Quiet moments of introspection in normal conversation may create many anxious ones for the patient, who cannot perceive the nonverbal aspects of silences and may wonder if he is expected to say something or whether he has already said something wrong. Worse yet, the nurse may be carrying on a private conversation about him by nodding and gesturing toward someone outside his door. There is also the unpardonable possibility that the nurse has quietly left the room without telling the patient.

Sometimes the patient may give the impression that he is hard of hearing. Because he may be unable to judge the distance between himself and more than one individual in his room, he may speak in a "broadcast voice."[17] Like a loudspeaker, his voice fills the room to reach the person who addressed him. In fact, in the public's mind, deafness is often seen as a natural sequela to blindness. With impeccable poor taste, some people address the blind individual through a third person. "Ask him if he would like a chair" or a similar comment has become almost classic.

Given time, the patient's "most influential impressions will be gained from the voices of others."[18] Just as we can surmise from a telephone conversation the sex, attitude, and approximate age of a caller, the blind person learns to evaluate moods and emotional responses. By listening with great acuity, he may detect the restless sounds of fidgeting and the rapid respirations of tension. Touch can also give him some information about the speaker. He can "feel human emotions by the shake of a hand" or by holding on to the nurse's arm.[19] Although the patient may come to know his environment by touch, he does not like to be touched any more than does a sighted person, and he has no desire to "feel by touch the facial features of others."[18] Common courtesy requires that the nurse identify herself and others in the room and explain the reason for touching the patient before doing so.

Nursing intervention. The individual who loses his sight is besieged by a host of psychic numbings. The core of his security has been shaken. One of the highest priorities for the entire health team is intervention that helps such a patient to regain a sense of stability. Daily assistance in replacing lost skills with new ones helps him to become cognizant of the ways to live a full life without sight.

Cardinal to a sense of safety is orienting the patient to the everyday sounds in the environment: the meaning of the various buzzers and the squeak of the medicine cart. He should never be left alone where sudden and unfamiliar noises may scare him. Background sounds unattached to symbols create frightening foregrounds. Knowledge that help is available when needed is critical to feeling safe. A call bell secured somewhere within his reach can substitute for a call light. The patient should have some indication when a conversation is ending and when the nurse leaves the room. To prevent him from being startled and startling others, the patient should be alerted to turn on the light rather than sit in a darkened room.

For the patient to accept his new body image, others must accept him. Keeping the patient abreast of current events relieves his feelings of being cut off from the world. Conversation that flows naturally communicates that he is a normal human being. Conspicuous efforts to avoid the words *see, look,* and *watch,* only cause embarrassment for both the patient and nurse. "See what I mean," "Now look what I did," and "Watch out" are customary ways of saying, "Do you understand?" "How clumsy of me," and "Be careful."

Security needs are also met when the patient learns to manage his meals. In privacy the patient can experiment with the setup on his tray, and whatever arrangement of food and utensils he selects should be used with continuity. Until the patient is able to feed himself, he should be privately and tactfully assisted. Nothing is more discouraging than bringing an empty spoon to one's mouth. The patient should be given a mental picture of his menu, as well as his environment.

Knowing where things are in his room strengthens the patient's sense of safety. In helping the patient explore his surroundings, the nurse should offer her arm to the patient and walk slightly in front of him. By mentioning approached hazards and alerting him when to stop and to step up or down, she diminishes the patient's fear of threats in front of him. His room should be as uncluttered as possible, and if something is moved the patient should be informed. Since a half-open door is hazardous, he should decide whether he wants it open or closed. Simply to close the door when one leaves makes him feel more isolated from the hospital community.

To become blind is to experience an avalanche of losses. First, the patient has to be supported into a system of human experiences in which there are no easy ways, only various hard ones. He needs to believe that in his making a new life adjustment the nurse will endorse his efforts to elaborate as a total human being. Within this emotional climate the patient may begin to consider various kinds of rehabilitation to make him feel more a part of life, rather than apart from it. Touch reading by coded raised dots, or Braille, and the use of a guide dog or special cane may help him regain self-approval and social autonomy.

Related to the increase in life span in this country is an increase in blindness, and many of the new cases yearly could have been prevented with our present knowledge.[20] The nurse needs to be aware that the primary means of prevention is the early recognition and prompt medical evaluation of all eye complaints.

Loss of hearing

Deafness is described as the "most desperate of human calamities" and a secular purgatory.[21] It causes the most profound depressions, and the "loneliness and isolation may lead to disorientation and a lack of desire to live."[22] Since deafness, like the invisible handicap it is, does not have the sheer number of losses as blindness, the manner in which it affects life is also less obvious.

Communication barriers. An undeniable loss is facility in interpersonal communication. Although people who cannot hear have been stigmatized as *deaf-dumb* and *deaf-mute,* they have the mechanism for speech and can use it with varying degrees of proficiency to communicate with the hearing. Like the patient who cannot see, the deaf patient must become aware of the nurse's presence before initiating conversation. Since he cannot hear the quality of his own voice, he may speak in a poorly understood monotone. Communication with the deaf patient can be established with patience and a little ingenuity. Most individuals become deaf at an age when they have some language skills, and "writing is the most used and most reliable method employed by the deaf" when faced with new situations.[23]

By keen observation and intelligent synthesis the patient may be able to understand the nurse's conversation by speechreading. In speechreading, formerly called *lipreading,* the patient makes use of all the visual aspects of communication: mouth and jaw movements, facial expressions, posture and gestures.[24] Since only one third of the sounds of words are visible, successful speechreading is contingent on many environmental factors. For example, the nurse's face must be adequately lighted. If the light is behind her head, it will cast shadows over her face and glare into the patient's eyes. The nurse should have nothing in her mouth. Using simple sentences, she should speak to the patient in a quiet, natural manner and pace. Speechreading depends in part on intelligent guessing. Helpful to the patient are such situational clues as introducing topics and showing pictures or symbols that represent treatments or procedures. Although speechreading requires the attentiveness of both participants, it can be extremely fatiguing to the patient. Not only must he interpret what was said but also formulate a response while continuously observing the nurse.

Alternate methods to writing and speechreading are available to patients with less verbal skill. One of these is sign language, in which the same techniques as those used to communicate with individuals who speak a foreign language are employed. Using the vocabulary of her body, the nurse can demonstrate or pantomime the ideas she wishes to express. If the nurse cannot "talk with the patient, at least talk to him," for the flux and flexibility of facial expressions and gestures that accompany words also transmit emotions that give many words their meaning.[25] Another technique of communication familiar to most deaf persons is finger spelling—an easily learned method of manipulating the fingers on one hand to coincide with the different letters of the alphabet.[24] Pictures of this manual alphabet may be obtained from any organization that works with the deaf adult.

The inability to hear is also compounded by the fear of being misunderstood. It is important from the beginning for the nurse and patient to recognize that they may not be able to understand each other but that the nurse will do her best to help him make his needs and intentions understood. Impatience may be an inevitable consequence of having to repeat the same communication several times. The patient may express his feelings of impotence by becoming obstinate and uncooperative. Chapman concluded that patients who are both "hostile" and "unintelligible" pose "the greatest threat" to helpers and are thus "subject to the strongest avoidance"[26] and social isolation.

Even though communication may be difficult, the deaf person can be aided in the use of compensatory techniques to offset some of the effects of his disability. Thus deafness need not constitute the most desperate of human conditions.

Let us turn now to hearing. Sight and hearing are senses that alert us at a distance to dangers undetectable by smell, taste, and touch. For survival purposes, sound has the advantage of bending around corners and traveling through dark buildings. The ears are always on duty; since there are no "earlids" to open and close, man is in a constant state of alertness to environmental threats. Hearing is unique because it can capture the sound of a distant siren, as well as the direction of the fire engine. The loss of hearing makes the individual more susceptible to threats behind him, and the fear of something overtaking him may contribute to the "reported higher incidence of paranoia among the deaf than among the blind."[27]

The deep depression of the deaf patient can cause disabling self-perceptions and misinterpretations of situations in his immediate surroundings. Whereas the blind patient has only a short pause in a conversation to fill with his fantasy, the deaf one has more time to improvise dialogue for a silent drama before him. A friendly talk between two student nurses outside the patient's door could bring his anxieties to center stage. Silent scenes are intensely penetrated by sight, and conversation in the patient's presence is sometimes thought to concern him. Intensely perceiving a situation by sight is staring, and eye contact begets eye contact. Hence the nurses would automatically return his glances. Should they continue to laugh and talk while doing so, the patient may think that derogatory remarks are being directed toward him. Anticipation of what may occur and a brief explanation if it does may help to allay some of the patient's suspicions.

All of us have emotional chords that whether accidentally or intentionally struck sound a discordant note. A hearing person whose entrance into the room terminates a lively conversation more than once will probably conclude that he is the target of criticism. One does not have to be ill to be hurt by a real or imagined wrong. The absence of sound does not create paranoid tendencies; we all have them.

In addition, the deaf person need not live a life looking over his shoulder. Just as some dogs have been trained to "see," others have been trained to "hear." Despite the significance of sound as warning signals, this loss does not have to constitute a calamity.

A cogent point is that the human brain is "equipped with something akin to sonar machinery" capable of picking up sound signals that change every second—the flutter of eyelids or falling raindrops.[28] The background sounds of changes in our bodies, such as heartbeats and joint movement, establish within us unconscious sensations of aliveness. When our body sounds couple with the background sounds of nature, we experience the "comfortable sense of being part of a living, active world."[29] When man can no longer hear, one of his most basic psychologic links to the world is missing, and this accounts for his overwhelming feelings of deadness. The individual who is born deaf has no such sense of loss because he was never aware of this "primitive level of hearing."[29] Deafness, then, can be the most desperate of human calamities because the individual feels dead for no *apparent* reason. Although diagnosing a condition does not cure it, the patient, at least, will know the nature of his complaints.

Comparisons to events in everyday life can often help the patient to cope with a new set of reality circumstances. That the undertones and vibrations of sound waves can give life a dynamic quality seems to be instinctively perceived by adolescents. They cannot understand why their parents insist that studying is impossible when the radio or stereo is blaring. Similarly parents often find contentment in the peace and quiet for the first few days their children are in camp, but by the end of the week they complain that "it sure is dead around here!" The nurse may be one of the most important figures in the patient's life during this morbid period. The time taken to enter into his system of communication supports and strengthens his ability to be alone with himself. Feelings of deadness may be diminished by dialogue with oneself. Communicating with oneself may help to convert the pathos of loneliness into the capacity to be alone. The capacity to enjoy solitude and engage in introspection or other kinds of creative activities makes one less reliant on interpersonal experiences for a meaningful and satisfying existence.

Partial loss of sight and hearing

Individuals with some functional sight or hearing may be "legally" classified as blind or deaf.[30] They are severely handicapped, but their handicap is not blindness or deafness but partial sightedness and hearing. Ironically, the individual with limited visual and auditory perception may have more problems in the presentation of self than do the blind or deaf.

Depending on state of health and such environmental factors as weather or noise, the individual with a partial sensory loss may be able to see or hear better on some days than on others. This confuses the public and humiliates the patient, who may feel compelled to give plausible answers even to his family. He is neither at home with the public nor comfortable with the totally handicapped. The latter may resent the individual who has poor eyesight or is hard of hearing because such individuals may account for spectacular case histories of adjustment and successful job placement. The person who has some capacity to communicate with eyes or ears is in social limbo. Most people have a poor understanding of the nature of this handicap and resist understanding what does not reinforce their opinions. Communicative approaches to the partically handicapped should help them use their abilities to the best advantage. This may soften the edge of having to validate themselves in terms of social mislabeling, rather than being allowed to find valid and useful that which society offers to some others.

Summary

Keeping the channels of communication open among members of the health team is important in all patient-care situations, but vital to the care of the patient with a body image problem. The patient will become discouraged from reiterating the same information and feel that he cannot depend on health care providers who do not communicate with each other. The road to reality is often difficult, and the individual whose body image has been radically altered has a great need to reminisce. The nurse may think that the patient is not making progress, but looking backward is more than regret for the past. It is part of a deep inner reference that gives the individual a sense of worth and the strength needed to reenter society.

Solitary contemplation is voluntary; solitary confinement is not. Although social rejection is not thought of as solitary confinement, there is little distance between the two points. We think of charity for the handicapped as virtuous human conduct but give little thought to human circumstances that often make charity a necessity. Preferable to the present climate is a converging of social concerns and actions that militate against treating the handicapped as second-class citizens.

OBESITY: GAIN IN BODY DIMENSIONS

Man's diversity is one of nature's greatest bequests. Ironically, this infinite variety in human beings makes it easy to convince oneself that one is better than someone else. The plump figures in Renaissance art show that man tends to create ideal body images reflective of social status and social acceptance at a particular time in history. A society that weighs personal potential in terms of physique encourages and perpetuates the stigmatizing of those who differ from the norm. Contemporary society would homogenize the human form into trim packages, and obesity is regarded with repugnance. Obese males, however, are not as socially handicapped as are females, and the color and design of their clothing tend to conceal excess poundage. Understandably, since feminine fashions accentuate the figure, females feel more compelled to seek some compromise between their human forms and the cultural ideals. Moreover, the obese male is usually described as *stocky*, implying muscles, and the female as *stout*, implying bulk.

The trend toward cultural unity makes it difficult for the overweight individual to maintain a sense of personal dignity. Coercive, cajoling messages from all the media promote health spas, fad diets, miracle pills, and exercising paraphernalia. This mass publicity and promotion eradicate personal excuses for being overweight. There are many ways to reduce if one has the will.

Excessive girth tends to be related to gluttony, which, as one of the seven deadly sins, is synonymous with an immoral lack of self-control. Stigmatizing the obese becomes sanctified by the puritanical abhorrence of self-indulgence. Whenever the stigmatized are believed to be the cause of their own condition, irrational attitudes toward them become exaggerated.[4] Some individuals seem committed to the flagrant enjoyment of another's failure, and, because the obese individual's body bears witness to his weakness, he may be ridiculed, avoided, despised, and discriminated against.[31] Society, like a fun-house mirror, magnifies problems, and this loathing from without can lead to self-loathing within.

Self-contempt can begin at an early age. Peer group behavior is essentially imitative of that found in adults but has the additional advantage of being authentic. Hence there can be no better pragmatic test of attitudes toward the obese than the practice of the young. It was found that among a heterogeneous group of children, some obviously disfigured and handicapped, the obese child was unanimously selected as being the most disliked.[32] When individuals grossly deviate from the desirable physique, many other imperfections may be fallaciously imputed to them.

Attitudes can obscure real issues while purporting to explain them but would not survive if they did not serve the psyche. Stigmatized individuals have low social status; therefore they are status builders for others. Degrading the obese makes certain individuals feel superior. By comparing their bodies to the obese, they "derive a modicum of self-esteem" with the additional advantage of "having social support for their own sense of status enhancement."[33] High status is believed to banish basic insecurities, and for this reason some individuals debase others to achieve it.

After a medical examination the obese person is usually told that there is no organic explanation for his condition and is not encouraged to believe that the medical profession is dedicated to finding one. On the contrary, one study revealed that some physicians regard the obese as "weak willed," "ugly," "awkward," and suffering more from malaise and lack of motivation than from a treatable medical disorder.[34] Because of the exclusion of physical evidence and negative attitudes toward the obese, the onus for overweight is the patient's by default. Social advocacy of the value of health and the relationship of excessive weight to such ailments as diabetes and cardiovascular diseases do not fully explain the social stance against obesity. Excessive smoking and drinking are as much a loss of ego control as is overeating and may be more detrimental to health; yet they are not uniformly regarded as social liabilities. Moreover, the "association of body fat and mortality below the level of frank obesity is not clear."[35] *Appearance,* more than the commonly promoted issue of health, may be the most plausible reason for negative attitudes toward the obese.

Although the etiologic factors in obesity are multiple, the role of inheritance may not be so minor. Many geneticists now think that recessive genes may be responsible for obesity and that the fat person is no more neurotic than is the normal or underweight person.[36] Constitutional predisposition may also exert a significant influence. Man inherits three basic body builds: *endomorphic,* or soft and round; *mesomorphic,* or muscular; and *ectomorphic,* or slender.[36] Ectomorphs may have longer and heavier intestinal tracts, and mesomorphs tend to have bigger muscles and bone mass. Recent investigations correlate excessive weight gain with the number of fat cells laid down in late fetal development and early infancy.[37] Overnutrition during these periods was concluded to predispose one to childhood and adult obesity; although dieting may decrease the amount of fat in each cell, the number of fat cells remains constant throughout life.

Another variable in obesity is the individual's level of physical activity and socioeconomic status. The person who gets little exercise may eat less than does the person of normal weight, but because of less energy expenditure, the unused calories are stored as fat. With a limited income, food choices are also limited, and the individual's diet may include greater amounts of filling carbohydrates.

Compulsive eating is common to the obese.[38] Associated with food addiction are other oral activities such as talking, smoking, gum chewing, and nail-biting. Such involvement with the mouth suggests that obesity may result from problems engendered in the oral stage of development.[39] The problem could be one of parental indifference or indulgence. The consoling "Don't cry; have a cookie," if consistently used, teaches the child to ingest a favorite food, rather than express an unpleasant feeling. Whatever the root cause, there tends to be a dissociation between eating and the satiation of physiologic needs. Instead emotional arousal becomes the basis for much compulsive eating.[38] Almost any emotion can translate into a need for food. Being unable to identify the emotion or his reaction to it, the obese person simplifies sensations as hunger. Feelings of loneliness or happiness can trigger overeating. Food is used for consolation and celebration. The obese rhapsodize about food, however it is used. They "love" pound cake, "adore" chocolate candy, and think banana splits are "exquisite." Symbolically food satisfies some unfulfilled need, be it for love or new experience.[39]

Like an alcoholic taking his first drink, the dieter can launch a binge with a single potato chip. The rationalization that "one can't hurt; it's only 15 calories" progresses to "oh, well, since I'm off the diet anyway, I might as well have another—and another"; but emotional gratification has guilt and self-hate as its feedback, and in a cyclic fashion these unpleasant emotions create the need for more overeating. Although overeating does not produce a state of intoxication, it can cause drowsy inertia. Food is soporific and temporarily relieves tension. During times of emotional deprivation, such as after being jilted, feeding rituals may be used to assuage depressive feelings. Conversely, weight loss is associated with falling in love; the fact that lovers are seldom hungry, no doubt, gives rise to the myth that two can live as cheaply as one. As with other habituation syndromes, when the obese's food intake is curtailed or restricted, withdrawal symptoms of irritability, weakness, indigestion, fatigue, and headache may occur.[38]

Virtually all obese persons have tried to lose weight, usually many times, and most are familiar with the latest methods of doing so. According to Buchanan,[36] the boundary between illusion and the reality of their body image is confused, and the obese tend to fantasize themselves as being free of defects. They misjudge body proportions and make mistakes in buying clothes, going through doors, and sitting in chairs. Because they nibble a great deal, they misjudge their food intake. This faulty perception may be due to training the eye not to see the body. Full-length mirrors and photographs are avoided; the face becomes the focus because it is the body area least distorted by fat. Depression may follow a rapid weight loss and is the reaction to a confused body image.[36] If the person grew up identifying himself as ugly and sloppy, a loss in weight means a loss of identity. The state of being unfamiliar with this new body may cause panic that can only be pacified by eating binges. Reducing calls for a compensatory revision in body image, without which the individual may oscillate in a "stuff-and-starve" cycle.

Some individuals must "cling to their girth" because unconsciously they feel that the layers of fat insulate them from the rebuffs of society.[40] They build mammoth body boundaries, which intimidate others and keep their own anxiety low. Reducing may be hazardous for the individual who sees no weaknesses in himself. Since fatness would no longer be an excuse for failure and self-hate, the individual's ego would be left defenseless against unresolved emotional conflicts.

The jolly fat man stereotype may be a thin disguise for deep anguish. The individual who has been insulted and scorned is unlikely to develop feelings of self-confidence and conviviality. However, given the choice between loneliness and participation in a group that may further deride him, the person may falsely present himself as a buffoon in preference to being excluded. In the presence of others he may joke and clown, although private feelings of isolation still permeate his existence. These private feelings become compelling reasons for attempts to escape from his corporeal prison. The inability to make further accommodations to social rejection is the principal reason for dieting.[41]

Hospitalization may be particularly humiliating. The obese patient may be unable to fit in the hospital gown, blood pressure cuff, or wheelchair. Two nurses may be needed to assist him in the routine activities of daily living. His weight may be measured on a special scale and his food intake carefully monitored. There will be little chance of concealing his body during routine examinations and treatments. He may initiate superficial dialogue, trying to disguise his embarrassment with good-natured levity.

Until more is known concerning the cause of obesity, the most humane approach would seem to be to regard the condition as a habituation syndrome. As in the treatment of other forms of addiction, multiple therapeutic approaches may be beneficial if the patient is not pressured or manipulated in accord with values of the staff. Exhorting the patient to stick to his diet and showing impatience and irritation when he fails to do so defeats the objectives of the nursing process. The patient then knows that the nurse respects neither his present self nor his potential to change. Acceptance is a prerequisite for healthy growth in relation to self and others and often for weight loss, but the latter must remain each person's prerogative. A cultural code that exacts physical conformity as a condition for belonging comes perilously close to denying the individual right to respond in one's own singular and special way.

If genuine interpersonal relationships are to occur, we must penetrate the surface of appearances. To do this we need to search our own vast repository of subjective references in which our prejudicial attitudes were schooled. Nursing intervention is inadequate unless we understand and help the patient to understand the reasons for some of the negative reactions he may face. Although obesity may complicate life, it should not determine it. We all are not beautiful, but we all are human beings. To analyze the cultural cliché that *beauty is only skin deep* is to conclude that the opposite also obtains: so are visible imperfections.

REFERENCES

1. Carroll, J.: Blindness, Boston, 1961, Little, Brown & Co., p. 1.
2. Ramsdall, D.: The psychology of the hard-of-hearing and the deafened adult. In Davis, H., and Silverman, A., editors: Hearing and deafness, New York, 1961, Holt, Rinehart & Winston, Inc., p. 462.
3. Macnamara, M.: Family in stress: social work before and after homotransplantations, Social Work **14**:95, 1969.
4. Kalisch, B.: The stigma of obesity, American Journal of Nursing **72**:1124-1127, 1972.
5. Fisher, S., and Cleveland, S.: Body image and personality, New York, 1968, Dover Publications, Inc., p. 111.
6. Wade, M.: Immobility: effects on psychosocial equilibrium, American Journal of Nursing **67**:794-796, 1967.
7. Fisher and Cleveland, op. cit., p. 55.
8. Kneisl, C., and Ames, S.: Mental health concepts in medical-surgical nursing: a workbook, St. Louis, 1974, The C. V. Mosby Co., p. 46.
9. Mereness, D., and Taylor, C.: Essentials of psychiatric nursing, St. Louis, 1974, The C. V. Mosby Co., p. 291.
10. Ibid., p. 289.
11. Simmel, M.: On phantom limbs, Archives of Neurological Psychology **75**:637-647, 1956.
12. Santopietro, M.: Meeting the emotional needs of hemodialysis patients and their spouses, American Journal of Nursing **75**:629-632, 1975.
13. Rubin, R.: Body image and self-esteem, Nursing Outlook **16**:20-23, 1968.
14. Tourkow, L.: Scientific proceedings; psychic consequences of loss and replacement of body parts, Journal of the American Psychoanalytic Association **22**:176, 1974.
15. Rosenbaum, J., and Rosenbaum, V.: Conquering loneliness, New York, 1973, Hawthorn Books, Inc., p. 66.
16. Seeman, V.: Your sight, Boston, 1968, Little, Brown & Co., p. 6.
17. Cutsforth, T.: The blind in school and society, New York, 1951, American Foundation for the Blind, Inc., p. 204.
18. Lowenfeld, B.: Our blind children, Springfield, Ill., 1969, Charles C Thomas, Publisher, p. 84.
19. Ibid., p. 180.
20. Shafer, K., Sawyer, J., McCluskey, A., Beck, E., and Phipps, W.: Medical-surgical nursing, St. Louis, 1975, The C. V. Mosby Co., p. 818.
21. Wright, D.: Deafness, New York, 1969, Stein & Day Publishers, p. 5.
22. Shafer, Sawyer, McCluskey, Beck, and Phipps, op. cit., p. 627.
23. Furth, H. G.: Thinking without language, New York, 1966, The Free Press, p. 10.
24. Bender, R.: Communicating with the deaf, American Journal of Nursing **66**:757-760, 1966.
25. Muecke, M.: Overcoming the language barrier, Nursing Outlook **18**:53-54, 1970.
26. Chapman, J., and Chapman, H.: Behavior and health care: a humanistic helping process, St. Louis, 1975, The C. V. Mosby Co., p. 140.

27. Carroll, op. cit., p. 291.
28. Wilentz, J.: The senses of man, New York, 1968, Thomas Y. Crowell Co., p. 189.
29. Ramsdall, op. cit., p. 464.
30. Carroll, op. cit., p. 311.
31. Maddox, G., Back, K., and Liederman, W.: Overweight as social deviance and disability, Journal of Health and Social Behavior **9:**287-298, 1968.
32. Richardson, S., Goodman, N., Hastorf, A., and Dornbusch, S.: Cultural uniformity in reaction to physical disabilities, American Sociological Review **26:**241-247, 1961.
33. Allport, G.: The nature of prejudice, Garden City, N.Y., 1958, Doubleday & Co., Inc., p. 349.
34. Maddox, G., and Liederman, V.: Overweight as a social disability with medical implications, Journal of Medical Education **44:**214-220, 1969.
35. U. S. Public Health Service, Division of Chronic Diseases: Obesity and health, Publication No. 1485, Washington, D.C., 1966, U.S. Government Printing Office, p. 6.
36. Buchanan, J.: Five year psychoanalytic study of obesity, American Journal of Psychoanalysis **33:**30-41, 1973.
37. Taitz, L.: Infantile overnutrition and possible ill effects, Nutrition **26:**341-346, 1972.
38. Swanson, D., and Dinello, F.: Severe obesity as a habituation syndrome, Archives of General Psychiatry **22:**120-127, 1970.
39. Bruch, H.: Psychological aspects of overeating and obesity, Psychosomatics **5:**269-274, 1964.
40. Friedman, A.: Fat can be beautiful, New York, 1974, G. P. Putnam's Sons, p. 32.
41. Ibid., p. 78.

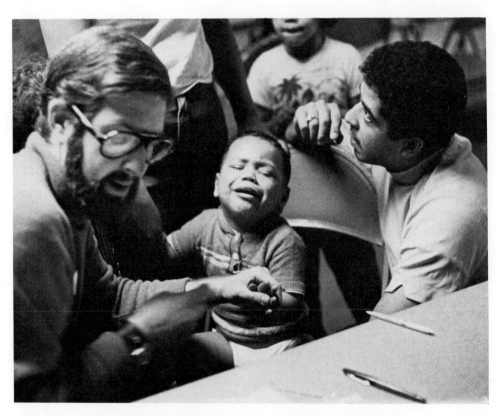

Chronicles of human life may be full of hurts—and healing. Some cries for compassion are more readily communicated than others. Pain and suffering are deeply personal—seared into the state of each person's inner being. If personal agony is to be eased, the healing process must be approached with *humility*, to delay assigning values to measures that seem evident—before reflecting on the meaning of *dignity*. (Photograph by Bruce Anspach, Editorial Photocolor Archives.)

CHAPTER 7

How shall humaneness in human relationships be defined: euthanasia and abortion

Conflict is characteristic of the human community. There are basic social and spiritual issues of life about which the most rational people will disagree. In the delivery of comprehensive health care the nurse needs to join representatives of other disciplines and members of the community in a search for solutions to critical issues confronting our society. A concerted and collegial effort is essential to fundamental fairness in communicating with individuals involved in two of the foremost issues today: *euthanasia* and *abortion.* Perhaps fittingly, this part of the text ends with a discussion of issues that bring us face-to-face with the complex meaning and value of life at the opposite ends of the continuum. In exchanging ideas, examining our ethical positions, and giving nursing care, we may help to improve our expertise in the art and science of communications through applying some of the concepts presented in the previous chapters.

THE CODE FOR NURSES

Intrinsic to the nursing process are issues of death and dying. Let us now consider standards of ethical conduct that relate specifically to these issues.

In nursing as in other professions, clarification and communication to practitioners of the desirable goals and normative standards of conduct to which members collectively subscribe are sought. In the "Code for Nurses" these values were formalized into ethical principles governing nursing practice, conduct, and relationships.[1] By publicly enunciating a unified value system, those in the profession affirm that they can be depended on to fulfill their social purpose. Inherent in the success of any human service is validating the public trust invested. The greater the trust, the greater the responsibility of professionals to enforce or defend their standards.

Science cannot be stayed. Man may soon be able to change his genetic

makeup, fertilize human eggs in the laboratory for implantation into
infertile women, and link the human brain to a computer.[2]

Each medical advancement seems to mandate a reevaluation of moral
responsibilities. Therefore the "Code for Nurses" cannot prescribe precise courses of action for each specific patient-care situation. Codes can
serve only as a basis for response and rational self-guidance in circumstances that do not involve clear, self-evident moral choices. Essentially
the nurse is expected to implement the ethics that she inherits as a
member of the profession. She is expected to do so not because the code
is infallible but because conduct compatible with the code seems prerequisite to making ethical decisions and discharging responsibilities to the
public, to other members of the health team, and to the profession.[1]

The following standards of conduct and interpretive statements ex-
cerpted from the code illustrate professional expectations that, as far
as the nurse's knowledge and competence permit, she will be responsible
for providing the patient with quality, individualized care and for protecting him from practices that threaten his health, welfare, or safety.
As a moral agent of the profession *the nurse has an obligation to—*

1. . . . provide services with respect for human dignity and the uniqueness
   of the client unrestricted by considerations of social or economic status,
   personal attributes, or the nature of health problems. Each client has the
   moral right to determine what will be done with his/her person; to be
   given information necessary for making informed judgments; to be told
   the possible effects of care; and to accept, refuse, or terminate treatment.
   . . . be knowledgeable about and to protect the moral and legal rights
   of all clients under state laws and applicable federal laws.
   . . . respect the worth and dignity of the individual human being irre-
   spective of the nature of the health problem. Concern for human dignity
   and the provision of quality nursing care is not limited by personal attitudes or beliefs. If personally opposed to the delivery of care in a particular
   case because of the nature of the health problem or the procedures to
   be used, the nurse is justified in refusing to participate. Such refusal
   should be made in advance and in time for other appropriate arrangements to be made for the client's nursing care.
   . . . protect the basic human values of the dying person while working
   with the client and others to arrive at the best decisions dictated by the
   circumstances, the client's rights and wishes, and the highest standards
   of care. The measures used to provide assistance should enable the client
   to live with as much comfort, dignity, and freedom from anxiety and pain
   as possible.
2. . . . safeguard the client and the public when health care and safety are
   affected by incompetent, unethical, or illegal practice of any person.
   . . . be alert to take "appropriate action" regarding any instances of incompetent, unethical, or illegal practice(s) by any members of the health care
   team or health care system that is prejudicial to the client's best interest.
3. . . . assume responsibility and accountability for individual nursing judgments and actions.[1]

An incident cited by Silva[2] is an excellent example of "appropriate action." A physician prescribed heavy doses of a tranquilizing drug to be given every 4 hours to a patient dying of cancer. Subsequently the drug produced the potentially lethal effect of a severe drop in blood pressure. In her role of patient's advocate, Silva directly communicated her concern to the physician, and the mutual goal of relieving the patient's suffering was achieved through a simple compromise: the drug was administered prn (whenever necessary) instead of every 4 hours. Appropriate action is deliberative action that is well thought about and through and based on objective analysis of what one wishes to accomplish and the implications of the decisions made to accomplish the goal.

The nurse's primary commitment, according to the code, is to the patient's care and safety. Human life should be respected, affirmed, and protected. The nurse has simultaneously a duty to help and perhaps an even greater duty not to harm. She is challenged to treat each patient according to his unique needs with justice, esteem, and dignity. Achievement of these human ends in patient-care situations of euthanasia and abortion seems contingent on respect for the human rights of recipients and providers of care.

Obligations outlined in the code may also conflict with the nurse's personal values of what is morally right or desirable and wrong or undesirable. Elective termination of pregnancy seems consistent with the value of giving nursing care according to the unique needs of the individual. The issue becomes complicated, however, with the question of whether one is caring for *one* patient—the mother—or *two* patients— the mother and fetus. In the latter instance the disagreement centers on establishing nursing priorities in patient-care situations involving competing rights. The nurse needs to ask herself what is the most responsible and equitable moral policy when values concerning human life conflict with values concerning human choice.

The ethical complexity and moral ambiguities in the issues of euthanasia and abortion may hold a permanent mortgage on our mental well-being. Questions concerning the quality and value of human life posed in an era of philosophic pluralism may never be answered to the satisfaction of all. Indeed, some may be unanswerable. Although it is impossible to specify in a code every type of situation that may be encountered in professional practice, directions and suggestions in the code may help resolve conflict over changing values within the profession and society. Because of the lack of consensus for any one absolute value, there are no easy remedies for moral problems. Another difficulty is that the code is externally derived and may lose meaning for, or be misinterpreted by, the individual practitioner.

Since the code cannot delineate precise nursing actions for specific situations, "the final test of ethical principles resides with the individual nurse's interpretation."[2] Coming to terms with some of the taunting ironies of real life requires *ethical reflection*. Ethical reflection opposes moral self-righteousness while exposing the subtle shadings of moral interpretations in each patient-care situation. Ethical reflection may help to distinguish between what is ignoble and what is human and between moral flaws and human frailties. Ethical reflection is a prerequisite to developing a personal code and humanely implementing the professional one.

Ethical reflection requires data gathering, which is contingent on effective communication. Dialogue with people holding contrasting points of view broadens one's perspective concerning a particular problem and is a necessary approach to understanding issues about which individuals differ. Although people may devoutly subscribe to diametrically opposed ethical positions, divergent personal and pastoral ethics do not necessarily equate with being uninformed or inhumane.

THE CONCEPT OF RIGHTS: BASIC HUMAN RIGHTS; NURSES' RIGHTS; PATIENTS' RIGHTS

In concert with rapid social changes, the health practitioner and the health care consumer have also changed. The consumer is becoming increasingly vocal in demands for quality health care. The tendency today is to define *quality care* in more than clinical terms. Although it may begin with efficient diagnosis and effective medical and surgical treatment modalities, the patient "generally defines quality care from a more humanistic point of view."[3] In this regard, the current concept of health recognizes rights in the area of humanness and respect for these rights in humane relationships. *Humanness* refers to whatever is characteristic of man and *humaneness* concern and compassion for him. When something is claimed as a right, the implication is that something is owed or due an individual. The consumer of health care is demanding as a just claim that health services have incorporated measures that support psychosocial integrity, and not just the treatment of diseases and infirmities. The patient wants sufficient information to enable him to make informed choices concerning his care and health services delivered in a respectful and dignified manner.

Basic human rights

In essence, individuals are seeking recognition of their basic human rights. Philosophically, basic human rights include privacy and security in what is most intimately one's own: body, intellect, spirit, family relationships, and personal possessions. Inherent in this is the right to self-determination and freedom of choice in life-style as long as one does not infringe on the rights of others. Basic human rights are the expression of feelings, inclinations, compassions, sympathies, intelligence, and thoughts.[4] This is simply a restatement of the need for therapeutic communication and to accord individuals the right to provide input into decisions that affect them. The lack of fulfillment of basic human rights has led to the drafting of many documents by and on behalf of various groups in their conscious efforts to be treated like human beings. The best-known statement regarding patients' rights was issued by the American Hospital Association in early 1973.[5] Primarily directed toward physicians, the document formally recognizes that a personal relationship is necessary for the proper provision of medical care. The latter includes the right to information, to give informed consent to or refusal of treatment, and to confidentiality. There are several such documents now in existence. The nurse needs to be familiar with the specific one adopted in the health care setting in which she is employed. These documents not only recognize the patient's right to humanitarian care but once adopted as policy may be legally enforced.[6]

More applicable to nursing practice than are medical and institutional policies may be the nursing process. Patients have a *right to the nursing process*. Through this process, nursing professionals seek to fulfill their social contract with consumers of health care. The nursing process promotes high regard for individual uniqueness, freedom of choice and the right to human dignity and justice and to make decisions for oneself. This process is central to therapeutic communication, which is central to the concept of humaneness.

The nursing process does not require the nurse to sacrifice her ethical principles. One who because of her religious background believes that the ending of a life is an unjustifiable means, however desirable the end, should exercise her right to remain uninvolved. Noninvolvement is a matter of self-respect and respect for the patient.

Nurses' rights

There is a direct correlation between human rights and nurses' rights. The nurse is first of all a human being and probably could not meet the requirements of ethical reflection and therapeutic communication if she herself felt unfairly treated as an individual.

The resolution on nurses' rights proposed by the Michigan Nurses' Association has become the model now used in the United States. Each right may be prefaced with the words "Be it resolved that . . ."

1. The nurse practitioner has the responsibility to inform employers, present and prospective, of her educational preparation, experience, clinical competencies and those ethical beliefs which would affect her practice.

2. The nurse practitioner has the responsibility to alter, adjust to or withdraw from situations which are in conflict with her preparation, competencies and beliefs.
3. The employer shall provide the resources through which health services are made available to the recipient.
4. The nurse practitioner has the right and responsibility to collaborate with her/his employer to create an environment which promotes and assures the delivery of optimum health services.
5. The nurse has the right to expect that her/his employer will respect her/his competencies, values, and individual differences as they relate to her/his practice.[7]

The five resolutions are similar to the code in that the first three statements focus more on responsibilities or obligations than on rights, or prerogatives. Familiar to most nurses is the second resolution, which to some extent rephrases the right *not* to do, or to refuse to participate. Equally significant, however, are the *positive assertions* of nurses' rights as human beings and professionals. From a combination of the ideas of Fagin[4] and Paulen,[8] one may conclude that the nurse has the following rights:

1. To *create an interpersonal relationship with patients*—to participate freely and effectively in planning and implementing care and to have her contributions respected and recognized with proper professional and economic rewards.
2. To *be authentic in her feelings.* Authentic feelings are the inner core of emotional and self-security. Ignoring feelings may lead to self-alienation and insensitivity. Recognition and acceptance of feelings helps one to assume the attendant responsibility for handling them.
3. To *find dignity in self-expression*—to be heard, to question, to doubt, to have no answers, and to err. In seeking to make reasoned ethical choices, the nurse has the right to receive support from others in the form of listening—sharing and caring—the right to an outlet for her frustrations and fears.
4. To *a work environment that minimizes health risks*—to have her strengths and weaknesses as a human being recognized and to be relieved of continuously working in patient-care situations in which tension, anxiety, and depression may be a consequence of confronting seemingly insoluble moral issues. Quality care depends on the nurse's general well-being. To expect the nurse to deliver quality care when her own physical and mental resources are depleted is unrealistic.

Rights are based on reciprocity of respect—allowing others, patients and professional colleagues, the same freedom of choice that we assert for ourselves. This seems essential to collaborative efforts to implement the nursing process as humanely as possible.

The dying person's bill of rights

Some rights have been refined to cover groups of patients with commonalities of care. The rights of the patient living his final human experience are indivisible from basic human rights and patients' rights because implicit in the latter sets is the belief that man experiences life as a unified whole. His physiologic, psychologic, social, and spiritual experiences inhere in all his responses to crises and the efforts that he makes to maintain personal integrity. The principles in the nursing process are just as applicable to the dying person as they are to any other living human being. The principles are modified and adapted to help the dying patient achieve his rights and to meet the requirements of his life situation.[9] He and those who love him have a right to the nursing process carried out in a climate of trust, sharing, sensitivity, and respect.

Trust links together all the phases of the nursing process in any human relationship. But life-threatening circumstances increase a person's dependency needs and reliance on health professionals. Bonds of trust thus become more than links in the nursing process; they are the bulwark on which it is based. The dying patient has a right to express his feelings and emotions about his approaching death in his own way and to have his questions answered as honestly as possible. Mistrust is a barrier to spontaneous expressions of true thoughts and feelings. The patient who mistrusts is unlikely to share his perceptions about changes in his condition, to ask the heartfelt questions that are really on his mind, or to consider plans for the future of his family openly. This kind of information can be obtained only through therapeutic communication. Close attention to the patient's verbal and nonverbal behavior is extremely important if the nursing process is to be kept current with his needs.

The dying person has a right to retain his individuality and not to be judged for decisions contrary to the beliefs of others. Sensitivity to the concept of wholeness supports the patient's right to uniqueness in human responses. Significantly, self-acceptance is a corollary to trust. The nurse who accepts herself may be more at ease with persons whose human values and coping mechanisms are unconventional. There is also the likelihood that she will listen to ideas alien to her way of thinking without communicating the conviction that she knows what is best.

The dying patient has a right not to die alone, to be free from pain, and to be cared for by knowledgeable, caring persons who will attempt to understand his needs. With changes in the patient's condition, priorities in the nursing process may also change. The plan of care is ever evolving. A mutually trusting partnership must extend to peers and encourage their contributions to the nursing process. In a genuine partnership the rights of significant others to make responsible choices with the patient regarding his care or on his behalf when he is unable to do so are also respected.

Caring for the dying person as a unique individual requires ethical reflection, which may help the nurse to clarify the distinction between the quality of living and the quality of dying. This distinction is important in seeking a personal answer to the ethical questions of what the proper respect for the needs of the patient and his family is when treatment of the sick becomes care of the dying and whether, when there is no prospect of reversing the ravages of disease or injury, the patient should not be allowed to die naturally at his own pace in the midst of his family instead of separated from them by mechanical devices? Respect for the rights of the terminally ill may mean that the practice of the art of healing becomes subordinate to the practice of the art of dying—that comfort, instead of cure, becomes the priority. Doing everything possible up to the last moment may obscure the dying person's needs, including the need to die, and deny him his right to a dignified death. By attending to his dying needs, we may better help him to be a part of life as long as he is with us.

Although the physician decides what treatment will best benefit the patient, the latter may also be benefited if the physician, nurse, clergy, and other members of the health team sit down to discuss how they may more effectively work together, implementing the bill of rights, so that the dying person feels cared for and about.

Some rights are more difficult to fulfill than others. The rights of the dying person may be among the hardest to bring to reality because dialogue about death symbolizes personal danger. In varying degrees, all of us have some fear or at least concern about death and a need to deny death. When one constantly confronts it, elaborate defenses against the idea of personal mortality are likely to be eroded. A normal reaction is to escape and minimize personal risk. When physical withdrawal is impossible, superficial dialogue and stereotyped responses may substitute for deep communicative involvement. Implementing the dying person's bill of rights may be an emotional ordeal. The nurse is under simultaneous pressure to cope with intrapsychic conflict, care for the dying person, and console and communicate with his family, with whom there is rarely any good news to share. Quint,[10] in her research on the care of the dying person, concluded that how the patient and his family live the last stages of his life is greatly influenced by the attitudes of the professionals caring for him. Kübler-Ross recommended that one

have respite to replenish emotional resources away from the presence
of death. Planned periods of withdrawal or periodic rotation to less
threatening health care settings implement the nurse's right to relief
from unremitting stress, which causes disequilibrium and discourages
the kind of sensitivity and ethical reflection needed for making considered
moral choices and for the humane discharge of the dying person's bill
of rights.

EUTHANASIA

The term *euthanasia* is of Greek origin and literally means good death.
The most frequently used English equivalent is *mercy killing,* meaning
that in certain circumstances, such as the presence of intolerable pain,
one may assist a person to a gentle, easy, and painless death. The
contemporary concept of *euthanasia* is the act or practice of "bringing
about the death of another for humanitarian reasons."[11]

Definitions of death

To ask what death is may not be so cynical as it seems. Currently
there exists no universally accepted definition of *death.* The traditional
legal definition is "the final and irreversible cessation of perceptible
heartbeat and respirations"[12]; as long as any heartbeat can be perceived
by any means and regardless of how it is maintained, death has not
occurred. This age-old criterion of clinical death lags behind such medical
advancements as the ability to sustain vital processes artificially.

Beauchamp points out that in the medical and nursing professions
two other types of death—cellular and biologic—are recognized.[11] Cellular
death is the irreversible degeneration of the individual cells, which may
precede or follow death of the rest of the body. Biologic death incorporates
the concept of "brain death," or state of damage from which the whole
person cannot be revived. Brain death, in this sense, is not the total
loss of brain function, but only the loss of cerebral function, or the
operation of the synthesizing mind, which determines that brain death
has ensued.[11]

However, this definition of *death* poses problems. When the cortical
brain cells that control such human capacities as communicating and
conscious body movements are damaged, the patient lapses into coma;
but this does not mean that the more resilient vegetative cells of the
midbrain or brain stem, which sustain automatic and unconscious
physiologic processes, are the only parts of the brain still functioning.
Although truly human qualities reside in the cerebrum, the conclusion
that with brain death the unique person also dies and becomes instead
a "vegetable" may not be entirely valid, for there presently is no "irrefut-
able objective evidence" for concluding that a patient is vegetatively

alive and cortically dead.[13] Sudnow[14] suggests that "nonresponsiveness" in the comatose patient may be the "inability to respond," rather than the inability to receive the stimulation. Since hearing is the last sense to disappear, perhaps in some instances the comatose patient may be cognizant of conversation around him but unable to let anyone know. Although the frequency is slight, some comatose patients classified as *hopeless* have been known to regain consciousness.[15] The concept of brain death creates an ethically troublesome dilemma: how to eliminate the possibility of error in determining the level and quality of life without needlessly prolonging the process of dying. What are the obligations to the comatose patient, who feels nothing, and to the family, whose pain and anguish grow deeper the longer the patient lingers? Prudent judgments will have to be made, and, in these kinds of patient-care situations, there may be no unanimous agreements.

With the advent of the possibility of heart transplants, an exact definition of *death* became urgent. In 1968 a statement of the World Medical Association and a report of an ad hoc committee of the Harvard Medical School agreed that death should be defined as irreversible coma or a permanently nonfunctioning brain.[16] Both documents listed four criteria signifying that a person is no longer alive, even though such physiologic processes as breathing and blood circulation are being mechanically maintained. Irreversible coma means (1) total unresponsiveness and lack of receptivity to external stimuli, (2) no spontaneous movement or breathing, (3) no reflexes, and (4) a *flat electroencephalogram* on tests made 24 hours apart. Proponents of this definition point out that establishing the moment of legal death is critical to the success of transplantation procedures. They believe that death is a complex process—that irreversible coma and evidence of a permanently nonfunctioning brain should be considered confirmatory evidence that the patient is dead, even though vital processes preventing clinical, organic, and cellular death are being artificially maintained. These vital processes therefore may be terminated for an organ transplant because concern over the four criteria of death protects the prospective donor from premature assaults. The fact that this definition has not yet been ratified by all the states may reflect societal concern for certainty. Euthanasia and death are inextricable. Variations in the definition of *death* may lead to varying opinions concerning what constitutes euthanasia.

Extraordinary means

Medical scientists have given man unprecedented means to prolong life by altering the natural outcomes of disease and trauma. At issue is the perplexing question that each nursing practitioner must answer for herself: "Is doing everything that can be done to preserve human life morally right?" Distinguishing between "ordinary" and "extraordinary" means may influence the nurse's answer, as well as her interpretation of intentional and unintentional killing. Pondering such questions and formulating tentative answers are necessary to the exercise of independent judgment and the provision of deliberative input into decisions about life and death.

No less a moral authority than the Pope seems to have voiced the view of major religions in stating that, "when life is ebbing hopelessly," the physician can limit ministrations to ordinary instead of extraordinary means "permitting the patient, already virtually dead, to pass on in peace."[17] Supporting the Pope's position, the Protestant theologian Paul Ramsey explains that, when a particular patient's dying has taken irreversible control, protection of life should not become useless torture, and respect for life should include respect for the dignity of the dying man.[18]

Concrete determination of what constitutes ordinary and extraordinary means independent of the circumstances in each case is difficult because the categories are relative and subject to change. For example, the insertion of a pacemaker several years ago may have been considered extraordinary, but today in areas of availability its use may be standard practice in the event of sudden heart block, as a safety measure after cardiac surgery, or in a medical illness that increases the risk of heart block. *Ordinary means* refers to normal food, drink, rest, and medical procedures "which offer a *hope of benefit* and which can be obtained and used without excessive expense, pain or other inconveniences."[19] Conversely, *extraordinary means* may be defined as all medicines and medical procedures "which cannot be obtained or use without excessive expense, pain, or other inconveniences for the patient or others, or if used *would not* offer reasonable hope or notable benefit to the patient."[20] Included under *extraordinary means* may be such artificial assistance of life as intravenous feedings, respirators, oxygen, blood transfusions, or chemical stimulants if there is no potential gain to the patient or if more harm than good may come from their use.

The concept of extraordinary means has been criticized on the basis that it is elitist: the use of a costly procedure may be ordinary for the rich but extraordinary for the poor. However, Smith[21] explains that the principle underlying the distinction is an attempt to "objectively define medical obligations" in terms of the total needs of the dying person and to acknowledge that need is highly variable.

Conceptually, extraordinary means may be thought of as "inappropriate to the circumstances."[22] In the delivery room, those in attendance are prepared to resuscitate immediately the newborn who does not breathe spontaneously. Physicians and nurses who care for newborns must be skilled in a method of resuscitation. However, if the infant has anomalies indicative of absence of cerebral tissue (anencephaly), the tendency is to make only "the most cursory efforts at resuscitation or none at all."[23] Vigorous resuscitation may be considered extraordinary means, since good effects might be outweighed by a short, institutionalized existence on a vegetative level. Another value is frankly admitted to come into play: it is more humane, and hence appropriate, for the grossly deformed infant and the parents to treat the child as a stillborn than to instill life temporarily in an infant faced with certain death.

Inappropriate to the circumstances may succinctly be defined as intervention that invalidates the right of the patient's family to consideration in maintaining their identity, integrity, and dignity.

Classifications

Primarily, there are two major classifications of euthanasia, which are further subdivided. The forms of euthanasia may be summarized as follows.

VOLUNTARY (Patient participates in decision)		INVOLUNTARY (Decision made on patient's behalf)
Direct, positive, or active: an act of commission	Patient may be provided with means to bring about own death	Relative, friend, or health personnel take affirmative action to cause patient's death intentionally
Indirect, negative, or passive: an act of omission	Patient gives discretionary powers to others to terminate life in the event he is unable to request or participate in the act of euthanasia	Extraordinary means are withheld or withdrawn, and the patient is "let go" when efforts to defeat death seem futile

Inherent in the doctrine of voluntary euthanasia are the elements of choice, purposeful rationality, and freedom to hold one's body and personality inviolate. The practice usually involves a competent adult who seeks a painless and quick release from a hopeless process of personal degeneration.

The *voluntary* and *direct* form of euthanasia is chosen and carried out by the individual. It is comparable to suicide. Examples might involve the homebound patient who requests a family member to leave an overdose of medication nearby and the hospitalized patient who refuses blood transfusions or dialysis.

In *voluntary* and *indirect* euthanasia, the choice may be made during or in advance of a terminal illness. The patient chooses and invests in a representative the right to make a prudent estimate of what the patient would want if he could be consulted. In addition, the patient may formalize in a "living will" his request that no heroic measures be taken to prolong life and needless suffering in the event that he becomes dysfunctional from an incurable illness.

Legislative proposals by euthanasia societies are mainly concerned with securing legal consensus for the voluntary forms, based on the philosophy that a person can make a fully free and mature choice of death to impart a final meaning to life when it becomes humanly meaningless. The patient who chooses to die may wish to talk about highly personal matters. Quint states that "when patients aware of their coming deaths talk about peripheral topics, such as reminiscing about the past, students have little difficulty either in listening or engaging in repartee."[24] However, when the patient speaks of his desire to bring a close to his life and to discuss such central issues as whether he will have uncontrollable pain or be conscious at the end, communication can cause considerable discomfort to the nurse, especially if the patient openly discusses plans for taking leave of his family and the staff or inquires about the nurse's personal philosophy of death. Conversation can be extremely anxiety provoking because in essence the nurse is being asked to consider her personal mortality consciously; then, too, the patient who exercises his right to refuse treatment is also rejecting the widely held medical and nursing value of preserving life. The nurse may react with anger, as a defense against the anxiety aroused when her values arc openly challenged and against feelings of helplessness and personal vulnerability. The most human contribution that the nurse can make is to listen. We need not condone the patient's choice, but perhaps with eithical reflection, moral condemnation will be suspended.

Involuntary euthanasia lacks the element of patient participation in the decision-making process. Whatever action is taken on the patient's behalf is without his request or consent.

Involuntary and *direct* euthanasia includes actions such as administration of a lethal drug or injecting an air bubble into a vein. Also included may be the addition of a drug, such as sodium pentothal, to a continuous infusion, inducing an irreversible state of somnolence in a relatively short span of time. In a somewhat gray area is the prolonged administration of a drug such as morphine to relieve pain in the last stages of an incurable illness. The moment of death can be hastened because this drug may have a toxic effect on respiratory, salivary, and heat-regulating mechanisms.[24a] Whereas the direct administration of a life-terminating agent may be considered an intentional evil act with an evil outcome, the management of pain with potent drugs over a period of time is done with good intent, although unintentional hastening of death may result in critical terminal cases. Despite cynicism about the infamous road that good intentions pave, the latter practice does not violate the accepted standards of reasonable medical care. The aim is freedom from pain and suffering, which consumes energy and generates a great deal of anxiety. Because anxiety is also energy depleting, the pain-anxiety syndrome can overwhelm the patient's mental and physical strength, leaving him demoralized and exhausted. Pain may dominate his life and limit his interest in all else. Pain is the most personal of human experiences; no one but the patient can experience his pain. Artful administration of analgesics in terminal illness involves the patient in the management of his pain. His verbal and nonverbal communications help the nurse to discern his needs, so that the potency and frequency of drugs can be continuously adjusted to conserve his "physical, mental, and moral resources and his social usefulness as long as possible."[25] The eminent theologian Fletcher is of the opinion that acts of commission, or directly intervening to bring about an easy death, are morally no different from acts of deliberate omission.[26] The end, or purpose, of both negative and positive euthanasia is exactly the same—to bring about the patient's death. Furthermore, letting an individual die a lingering death, dehumanized, is harder to justify morally than taking positive, direct actions to help him avoid it. Refuting Fletcher, the renowned theologian Weber[27] contends that "letting the patient go" is ethically acceptable, whereas direct killing is not. There is an enormous difference between not fighting death and actively putting an end to life. Giving up attempts to prolong life in a terminally ill patient and concentrating on his needs as a dying person are fully compatible with respect for human life; but, when a human agent, instead of disease, is the immediate cause of death, even with the best of intentions, the practice is "logically part of the view that human life itself is not enough to warrant our respect."[27]

Admittedly, there may be only a thin border line between causing and allowing a patient to die—thin because, although the means may differ, the end is the same: the death of an individual. However, Smith cautions that the ethical distinction between the two types of euthanasia should not be abandoned—that no direct, affirmative medical intervention is needed if "we understand the dispensability (nonmandatoriness) of both extraordinary and ordinary means which are not remedies."[28]

A practice is not necessarily in the patient's best interest or an act of kindness just because it is achievable.

Smith's position may be not only ethically sound but also legally sanctioned. In a landmark decision on March 31, 1976, the New Jersey Supreme Court ruled that the respirator that had helped to sustain Karen Anne Quinlan's breathing for nearly a year might be removed.[29] An individual was said to have a right to privacy and to refuse further invasion of his or her person by artificial life sustainers in an incurable illness. Thus, acting as her guardian, her father could exercise her right to choose a natural death once the attending physician and an ethics committee agreed that there was no hope of Karen's regaining her capacity for cognitive experience.

Although technically applying only to New Jersey, the decision could set a precedent for courts across the country. To achieve a dignified death may require awareness "that to die is one way of being a human creature, and to be allowed to die a precious human right."[30]

Legal implications

Discussion of the legal implications of the practice of euthanasia has been deliberately delayed until this point. No external authority can substitute for sensitivity to the possible abuses of power in making decisions involving critical life-preserving issues. The very defenselessness of the dying person imposes a special duty of care.

Although making decisions about life and death is the physician's prerogative, problems for the nurse must be recognized because nurses may take part in actions or be aware of inaction that determines whether life is maintained. How should the nurse respond to a physician's order to "pull the plug" or turn off the current of a respirator that has been keeping a patient alive for days or months? Do the nurse's ethical and legal responsibilities to the dying person require that in the absence of formal hospital policy she question a physician's chart order not to call the code for emergency resuscitation? Of interest is the fact that in the Karen Anne Quinlan case no mention was made of the role of the nurse.

To be brief, one may say that in our society, laws are designed to mitigate human conflict, actual or potential. Negligence is the central concept underlying American "tort" law. *Tort*, meaning wrong in French, refers to an injustice done another person whether intentionally or unintentionally in breach of a legal duty.[31] Negligent conduct on the part of the nurse rarely involves willful intent. More often it is a breach of the legal obligation of reasonable care. The nurse, in short, is obligated to act in a reasonably prudent manner to avoid causing harm or injury to others. The "reasonableness" of her conduct is measured against the standards of her professional peers; if under the same or similar circumstances her peers would have acted as she did, no liability is imposed, even though the patient may have been harmed. The nursing student may be surprised to learn that in clinical activities she can be held to the level of performance of the competent licensed professional nurse and is personally liable should harm result to the patient in the performance of her duties.[32] The patient is believed to have a right to competent nursing care at all times.

As those in the medical profession move away from diagnosis and treatment to consideration of questions of life and death, society, through its laws, allows health professionals less autonomy in making judgments. According to Meyers,[33] a positive act undertaken with the *willful* intent to cause death, even for merciful motives, is expressly prohibited by criminal law, and the possiblity of liability and prosecution for homicide are ever present. Aiding or abetting a competent adult to commit suicide may be considered a criminal act or a civil liability if the aggrieved parties, such as the employing institution or survivors, bring suit. For acts committed for humane reasons to be considered illegal may be unfair. Perhaps the evolution of new standards regarding such agonizing decisions is needed; however, health professionals, for all their knowledge, are not presumed by law to have more expertise about who should live and who should die than does the laity. Regarding the refusal to commence or continue the ordinary medical treatment required to maintain life or extraordinary measures, such as the use of a heart-lung machine after a massive stroke, the legal interpretation is meager and would appear to be lenient with respect to both methods provided the element of consent is given due consideration.

The point to remember is that, when cases of euthanasia reach the courts, legal disposition will be based on specific facts, instead of hypothetical situations, and, so long as the nurse is not negligent, she is free to exercise her most prudent professional judgment in her care of the terminally ill. Because there are few right answers, the "reasonable man" axiom is the one most likely to be legally applied.

Standards regarding the practice of euthanasia change only through painstaking resolution of conflicting philosophic, religious, and social interests—the interests of health professionals and of the patient and his family but most importantly the collective interest of all who must face death in a similar way.[31] Contemporary man cannot forget some of the horrors perpetrated at Dachau and Buchenwald, among others, and is wary of setting standards possibly implying that some lives are more worthy of living than others. An edict about when death should come or at least the standard under which decisions concerning its coming should be made is one that the law in a free society leaves ultimately to the people.

THE ABORTION DILEMMA

In the past, social changes were sufficiently slow to allow for gradual adjustments in human relationships. Nursing is a human relationship, and, as with all prevailing relationships, the traditions on which it is based have to be reexamined in terms of present-day realities.

Rights of the pregnant woman

The supreme court ruling in 1973, reiterated in 1976, affirming the right to abortions extended the scope of our social contract. The 1973 ruling eliminated in the first 3 months of gestation, the time when most abortions occur, all restrictions on voluntary interruption of pregnancy except for licensing of the physician. Restated, this means that in early pregnancy the decision to abort is left to the discretion of the patient and her physician. Beginning with the fourth month of pregnancy the state can set restrictions. By logical extension of the first ruling, in 1976 the Court mandated that, since the state is forbidden to veto abortions in early pregnancy, it cannot give someone else the power of veto. Thus the state can neither require a wife to obtain her husband's consent for abortion nor impose "blanket restrictions" requiring parents' or guardians' consent for abortion in single women under 18 years of age.[34] Although they noted the importance of safeguarding marital relationships and supporting parental authority, in the former instance the justices believed that, when a husband and wife disagree on the decision to abort, the view of only one of the partners can prevail; since the wife is more directly and immediately affected by the pregnancy, the ultimate decision should be hers. In the latter instance, their reasoning was that, if safe abortions are denied minors by parental fiat, hazardous illegal abortion may flourish.

Under the "conscience clause," physicians, staff members, and sometimes even the entire staffs of private hospitals have the right to refuse to participate on the basis of their personal convictions.

In nursing, pregnancy has always been considered to be an interrelationship between two patients; hence the emphasis is on prenatal care and unremitting efforts to maintain optimal health for the mother and the new life. Although the supreme court decisions concerning abortion were efforts to strike a balance between the state interest in protecting life and the welfare of the pregnant woman, the rulings have deeply disturbed the American psyche. Health professionals who have the responsibility for carrying out abortion procedures are divided.

Remember Mauksch's and David's declaration that the nursing process is the profession's prescription for survival in this era of rapid social change and rising human expectations. This process is an instrument of human service, and one of its strengths is the problem-solving approach to making delicate and difficult decisions. Ethical problems seldom have clear answers or final solutions. To the extent that our decisions are ill informed or intemperate, we do not implement the nursing process or the principles of a free society very well. Consideration is needed for the belief that mandatory motherhood disregards the woman's spiritual and social need to space and choose the number of her children and compromises her right to dignity and privacy "in matters relating to marriage, family, and sex."[35]

Abortion and morality

Prior to the fourth month of gestation, the state has no substantive interest in making a determination about the morality of abortion, but the moral climate within the community decidedly affects the availability of health care facilities for abortion. If the predominant attitude is antiabortion, the legal aspects may be constantly challenged, and the unhappily pregnant woman may in desperation seek a solution to her problem elsewhere.

Moral attitudes usually have roots stretching well into the past. Formerly, traditional sex mores for females were goal-directed toward childbirth. Sex for pleasure was synonymous with "the sins of Eve," and their wages were marriage and pregnancy. Childbirth was a form of expiation for one's sins, and unwanted children demanded self-sacrifice and subordination of the woman's wishes. Female sexuality as being in accord with total health needs was neither then nor is yet creditable. The basic assumption is that the fear of pregancy discourages promiscuity or sinning; therefore, if abortions are difficult to obtain, sin somehow will be suppressed.

However, aside from lack of reproductive and contraceptive information, there are myriad reasons for engaging in unprotected intercourse. Contrary to the opinions of many, sex for pleasure alone is not of the greatest magnitude.[36] Pregnancies, like accidents, do not necessarily just happen; unconscious motivation may be a major factor. Pregnancy may be an attempt to gain parental attention, to hold the male in a relationship, to resolve a shaky female identity and allay homosexual anxieties, as well as to punish the male.[37] When the realities of pregnancy fail to meet the motivational fantasies, abortion may become the preferred option.

To a large extent, a "responsibility ethic" is deeply ingrained in our societal psychosocial structure. In essence, this ethic implies that individuals *ought to be* willing to accept the consequences of their actions. Personal freedom is an esteemed value. "You made your bed; now lie in it" restates the belief that a noteworthy ingredient in freedom is accountability. The prestige of this ethic is strong enough to stigmatize those who deviate. Breach of the ethic causes a strong adverse reaction, and the person may be discredited as a less-than-worthy human being. This reaction may be intensified by the belief that abortion is a blatant repudiation of the ideal of maternal love, as well as rejection of pregnancy as the natural fulfillment of the feminine role.

Stigmatization leads to feelings of depression, loneliness, and isolation. The isolation may be self-imposed if the woman inwardly respects the societal code and feels ashamed and disgraced by her transgressions. Few women, according to de Beauvoir, approach the abortion experience without misgivings, and in her heart the woman "often repudiates the interruption of pregnancy which she is seeking to obtain."[38] Because her natural tendency can well be to have the baby whose birth she is undertaking to prevent, "she is divided against herself."[38] Even though she has no positive maternal desires and does not consider abortion to be murder, still it cannot be considered a mere contraceptive technique, for "an event has taken place that has a definite beginning, the progress of which is stopped."[38]

Callahan makes the interesting point that ironically "there would not be an intense abortion debate had not society moved to a higher plateau of moral sensitivity."[39] The advocacy of "women's rights" is a tribute to the growing concern that women have been discriminated against and treated as second-class citizens. Complaints about the physical hazards and personal degradation of illegal abortions reflect heightened sensitivity to the fact that the option of abortion (legal or illegal) has been less readily available to some groups than to others and that competent medical care and personal dignity should be available to the poor and ignorant, as well as to the affluent and educated. The encouragement of parents to plan their families is a tribute to the social efforts to enhance the quality of family life, taking into account not only physical but also developmental psychosocial needs of each family member throughout life. Although these factors seem to support liberalized abortion laws, arguments opposing such laws also stem in part from heightened moral awareness. The drive to keep abortion laws restrictive can be seen as a tribute to the research being done to protect life in utero. One example is intrauterine transfusions given in the event of serious fetal and maternal blood incompatibilities. Of great significance also is the subtle awareness that all forms of human life should be given due consideration: a rational concern that stems in part from an abhorrence of the disposability of human life at the will of those who hold power in totalitarian regimes. In other words, the abortion debate seems to parallel the growth in moral consciousness.[40]

In consideration of the morality of abortion, one probably will not encounter such a paragon as a neutral observer. The issue seems to encompass three possible ethical positions: all abortions are bad, all abortions are good, and abortions may be good or bad depending on the circumstances. The nurse who believes that all abortions are bad may not be able to give therapeutic care to abortion patients. Similarly the nurse who believes that all abortions are good is not likely to do the kind of assessment or impart the information that encourages the pregnant woman to make a fully informed choice. In fact, the nurse's attitude may unwittingly bias the pregnant woman's decision. The patient who feels pressured into having an abortion may later suffer severe grief and depression, hating "those who urge her to seek what in her inner motivation she opposes."[41] Conversely, the nurse who believes that abortion may be good in some instances and not in others may consider a range of factors in the abortion experience, such as the patient's attitude toward pregancy, the socioeconomic situation, significant relationships, and the need for supportive services, without having an intense need to communicate either ethical position to the patient. In essence, such a nurse can give individualized, humanistic care.

Each practitioner must weave a moral path through the varying points of view, ever alert to the possibility that the path of least resistance is often habitual modes of thought and careful not to stumble over the stones of semantics, since both sides define terminology to slant value judgments in their favor or to suggest categories of thought. A few examples, such as those given below, should suffice.

ANTIABORTION	PROABORTION
Abortion is murder by appointment.	Abortion is a minor surgical intervention.
A curette is a surgical instrument of death.	A curette is a spoon-shaped instrument used in the practice of obstetrics for cleaning out the uterus.
Saline induction is a method of wanton slaughter or "pickling alive."	Saline induction is a scientifically and medically approved method of stimulating uterine contractions.
The organism resulting from impregnation is a human being.	The organism is a product of conception.

Although the statements define the same terms, the emotional undertones derived from their differing emphasis can be potent enough to polarize moral positions. Extreme positions prevent us from thinking objectively when we try to formulate humanistic responses to a highly debatable ethical problem.

Morally reconciling the right to abortion with the act of abortion seems to be especially difficult for two reasons. First, approval of abortion is thought to compromise seriously the secular safeguards in the Constitution of the inalienable right to life. *Ideologically* the basic premise of the law is that all forms of life must be protected and that helpless life especially must not be endangered without necessity. Second, the practitioner must *personally* define human life and then determine for *herself* or *himself* the point in gestation at which life is inviolate. Contingent on her or his responses may be the humane implementation of the nursing process in the care of the person having an abortion.

What is human life?

The question what is human life? has to be further subdivided for a more objective inquiry. First, we must try to assess in scientific terms when life begins; having done this, we face the difficult task of assigning a value to it.

In the process of neonatal development several stages could reasonably be designated as the beginning of a new human life. Only four stages—fertilization, segmentation, fetal development, and quickening —are selected because these events occur in part or entirely before decisions concerning abortion revert to the authority of the state. In this brief discourse, only the major characteristics of each stage will be discussed. Bear in mind, however, that proponents of the "right to life" believe that the moment of conception is decisive for conferring humanity because at fertilization the new entity receives all its genetic information.[42] A being with a genetic code is said to be in the process of becoming, as is all human life, whether fetal, infant, or adolescent; and since every new entity has potentials similar to those of every other human being, the right to be born should be respected and protected.

The union of ovum and sperm forms a unicellular structure, called a *zygote,* whose genetic makeup is new to humankind. Thus the potential to become a unique individual could occur at the moment of conception. Within a week, this zygote, which has become a cluster of rapidly dividing cells, has completed its journey down the fallopian tubes and has begun the complex process of implantation in the uterine wall. The organism, now called a *blastocyst,* has specialized cells that secrete into the maternal bloodstream a hormone inhibiting maternal menstruation, which would prove fatal to its existence.

Approximately 2 weeks from the moment of origin of the genotype, the germinating matter segments into a complex triple-layered entity those ectodermal, endodermal, and mesodermal tissue will give rise to organs and organ systems. However, if the mass of cells separates into two or three (or more) sets, identical twins (or triplets, etc.) may be formed at this time. Although the sets of cells may recombine into one embryo, the unique genotype resulting from fertilization cannot be said to be "irreversibly an individual until about the beginning of the third week."[43] Prior to this time, there may be two or more entities in one blastocyst.

Four weeks after fertilization, under the influence of the developing brain, the structure that will later become the four-chambered heart begins pulsating and propelling blood through microscopic arteries. After 5 weeks, all traces of organs and organ systems are laid down, and the embryo, now a fetus, begins to assume human form and function. From that time on, the thrust of development is toward growth and maturation of existing structures, rather than the creation of new ones.

By the eighth week of fetal development, electrical activity of the brain can be detected by an encephalograph, and the heartbeat can be monitored by the twelfth week with refined electrocardiographic techniques. The fetus is now capable of making reflex and spontaneous movements. Maternal sensitivity to fetal movements is called quickening, or feeling life. Quickening is usually perceived by the pregnant woman at 16 weeks' gestation, although women who have been pregnant before may become aware of the movements much earlier.

Another major milestone in fetal development is the twentieth week. Between the sixteenth and twentieth weeks the fetal heartbeat can be detected through the pregnant woman's abdominal wall by stethoscope. Although legally the age of viability, or capacity for extrauterine survival, is 28 weeks, a fetus "between 20-28 weeks of gestation has a 10% chance of survival" today[44]; so its delivery may be classified as premature and not an abortion. The legal definition of *viability* is not in complete accord with scientific advancements in modern incubator management and the medical evidence for opposing rules of viability.

Notable is the medicolegal difference attached to the fetus at different stages of development. A fetus aborted spontaneously or by intent prior to 4½ months' gestation does not require a birth, death, or stillbirth certificate, legal interment, or baptism and is treated as a pathologic specimen.[45] After this time, however, some form of documentation may be required by the states to give formal recognition to a "new life" in the official annals of society. This seems to indicate a sociocultural distinction between a previable and potentially viable life and supports the notion that the previable fetus—the fetus that could not survive outside the uterus—is not a "human being," although it may well be a part of the biologic continuum of humankind.

Science seems to be able to tell us only that from the moment of fertilization the potential for new life is always in the process of becoming—from implantation, segmentation, fetal development, quickening, and beyond. However, science cannot tell us what values are to be imputed to the developing new life. After due consideration of competing points of view, the nurse must look to her own conscience for the final answer regarding her nursing actions. If she believes that personhood is conferred at the moment of conception and that abortion is the taking of human life, the following discussion is not an attempt to persuade her to believe otherwise. However, the belief that the zygote is a *potential* human being is appropriate for further exploration.

We have no specific terminology for the loss of the fertilized ovum prior to or in the early phases of implantation. Is it contraception or abortion?

Approximately 10 million women in the United States use the contraceptive pill.[46] Reproductive biologists explain that the pill could be producing its contraceptive effect in a variety of ways, one of which is causing changes in the lining of the uterus in such a manner that the fertilized ovum cannot imbed itself.[46] Additionally the intrauterine device (IUD) may be more properly classified as an abortifacient than a contraceptive because the presence of this foreign body in the uterus may not only interfere with the implantation of the products of conception but also have a *toxic* effect on the implanted embryo.[46] The universally acknowledged preferable ways of preventing unwanted pregnancy may in reality be abortions on a wide scale. If personhood is assigned to the fetus before or shortly after implantation, use of the pill and IUD is a highly questionable moral practice.

Predictably some hold that humanness is established at the end of the second month of gestation or at the time that brain waves are discernible. This hypothesis seems consistent with one of the latest criteria of death—a flat encephalogram; yet one cannot overlook the fact that the fetus has other signs of life, such as a heartbeat and reflex movements. In addition, brain functioning is in the process of development. One may be on safer ground to concede that new life is present but on a vegetative level because the cerebral cortex, the source of human characteristics, has not completely differentiated. Both the problems of euthanasia and abortion pertain to defining what is meant by *human life*. Therefore, since life supports can be withdrawn at the end of the life cycle for humanitarian reasons, the same rationale may be appropriately applied to the beginning. Perhaps legal abortion in the early months of gestation could be thought of as providing a period of "grace" for the woman who in the realm of private decision cannot find within her the mechanisms for coping with the exigencies of motherhood at this time in her life.

Of major import is the finding that the pregnant woman does not usually identity the new life as a potential human being until the time of quickening.[47] Prior to her perception of fetal movements the new life is not a reality—not a child to whom she feels a moral bond. Hence the patient who has an abortion prior to quickening may not think of the procedure in the absolute terms of destruction of a human life. Interruption of pregnancy prior to the patient's personal detection of fetal life tends to be associated with minimal postabortal psychologic ill effects.

In regard to forcible conception, or instances in which pregnancy results from rape or incest, few object to the proposition that compelling a woman to bear the child of her ravisher is cruel and inhumane. More morally complex, however, are situations in which genetic counseling shows that, in the framework of existing data, there is a certainty or calculable likelihood that the fetus may be severely physically or mentally incapacitated because of hereditary defects or exposure to harmful drugs, dangerous amounts of radiation, or such viral infections as rubella. Because of the rapidly refined techniques of amniocentesis, after the fourteenth week of pregnancy, cells in the fluid surrounding the fetus may be removed and studied and the presence of gross chromosomal, as well as some other congenital defects, detected. The problem is complex because the choice of abortion must be made in the fourth or fifth month of pregnancy; besides being more dangerous, the procedure would take place after quckening and conceivably after the age of viability. Then, too, there is concern that methods for detecting abnormalities may one day be far in advance of corrective technqiues and that standards regarding which fetuses are to be born and which to "die before birth" may evolve that justify taking a life on the basis of varying human potential.

On the other hand, there is the view that the family who finds such alternatives to abortion as financial assistance, therapeutic and rehabilitative procedures and facilities, and social casework unavailable or unacceptable could make a responsible choice of abortion on the basis of obligations to the pregnant woman and other family members to preserve the integrity of the existing family unit and protect it from the emotional and social catastrophe that a grossly deformed newborn may precipitate.

Unwanted pregnancy: a medical disease?

A tremendous contribution would be made to the abortion debate if the current term could be replaced with a less emotionally charged word. The term *abortion* evokes unbidden, powerful attitudinal patterns of propriety and tends to draw needed attention away from other pertinent data. That idioms can advance ideologies is exemplified by the fact that when *family planning* became the euphemism for *birth control,* dialogue concerning the practice became more dispassionate and the public more favorably disposed. Pion, a physician, suggested that treating unwanted pregnancy as a disease would provide more objective structure to a series of salient facts.[48] Once a problem can be restated in neutral terms, it may be less likely to cause emotional distractions.

As an elaboration on Pion's proposition, unwanted pregnancy is further hypothesized to be a human health problem of major proportions, affecting the patient, her family, and the community. The concept of unwanted pregnancy may be brought into consonance with that of disease for the following reasons:

1. Regardless of their social characteristics, a large number of females of childbearing age are susceptible.
2. Progression of the disease can threaten the spiritual, mental, and socioeconomic health of the patient.
3. Significant established relationships may be disrupted or put at risk if responsibility for an additional member of the family is imposed.
4. The disease can be readily diagnosed.
5. The treatment is known, and the minor surgical procedures are relatively safe and inexpensive.
6. Physical and emotional factors contraindicating treatment can be discerned.
7. Trusted consultation and supportive services may render the disease "benign," or turn an unwanted pregnancy into a wanted one.
8. The nature of the disease and treatment can be frankly communicated to the pregnant woman for voluntary decision making.
9. Medical supervision is preferable to the hazards of self-treatment or intervention by unqualified practitioners.
10. The disease is preventable and ongoing, and follow-up care can be provided according to personal need.
11. The patient may be able to avail herself of treatment, based on sound health determinants, that she and her physician deem to be in her best interest.

A major criticism of the analogy between unwanted pregnancy and disease is the belief that the "tissue growth" within the woman's body is by no means part of her, as are her tonsils or other organs. Being only a "host" to the fetus, the woman cannot make decisions regarding it. Fetal tissue has a unique genetic makeup, fixed from the time of fertilization, and there will never be another mass of vegetating cells identical to it. The separate genetic constitution of the conceptus—its individual circulatory, hormonal, and nervous systems—distinguishes the new entity from its mother. Unless life supports are withdrawn or interfered with, this cluster of developing cells has the potential to develop into a person. The human potential of the tissue sets abortions apart from other minor surgical procedures.

Another obstacle to treating unwanted pregnancy as a disease is that major organic disturbances, such as cardiovascular and renal disorders, are eliminated as automatic indications for abortion because of present medical knowledge, conditions that pose a serious threat to the pregnant woman's well-being have been drastically reduced. Furthermore, in the early months of gestation the question whether to perform an abortion to save the life of the patient is moot. The choice, if there is one, is to do everything possible to save the patient or risk the death of the patient and the fetus, who is inexorably dependent on her.

Also excluded are the instances in which continued pregnancy would produce serious and permanent impairment of the patient's mental health in medicolegal terms. If the patient who becomes pregnant is floridly schizophrenic, psychotically depressed, or has had previous severe postpartum depression, carrying a pregnancy to term may constitute substantial risk to her mental health. Note also that in the area of less severe character disorders and neuroses, suicidal ideation "is one of the commonest" justifications for terminating pregnancy, although actual suicides under these circumstances are said to be rare.[49] According to Mecklenburg,[50] reasons for the low suicide rate may be twofold: first, "the woman receives more attention from society when pregnant than nonpregnant" and, second, "certain physiologic and instinctive factors which manifest themselves in greater maternal protectiveness" may be operant. This contention can be challenged, however, on the basis that the woman who seeks to end an unwanted pregnancy by putting her life in the hands of an illegal abortionist is in a strict sense courting death.

From this generalization, unwanted pregnancy would seem to constitute a major public health problem. The woman who is convinced that termination of pregnancy is the right course of action will risk criminal abortion at tremendous hazards to her safety. Data collection concerning the incidence and complications of illegal abortion may be unreliable because a successful abortion remains a secret. Moreover, when complications, such as infection, result, they may be privately treated with antibiotics. Lacking any real accuracy, statistics may be used to support or refute the position that unwanted pregnancy constitutes a major health problem. Figures cited on the frequency of induced abortions range from a low of 200,000 to a high of 1,200,000 each year and related deaths from 500 to thousands of deaths annually.[51] Yet, even if the lowest figures are closest to the truth, a fair conclusion might be that access to an abortion procedure that is relatively safe and simple when performed under proper conditions would eliminate or significantly reduce the toll of needless injury or death.

Although the concept of unwanted pregnancy as a disease has weaknesses, it represents a serious attempt to approach the abortion problem from a different perspective, which may be useful for ethical reflection. A good beginning may be to focus more attention on the father of the unborn child. Although he is an equal partner in the act of procreation, the selective social inattention that he receives leaves him virtually free to continue his life as he chooses. However, should he suffer one of the unfortunate side effects of copulation, such as syphilis or gonorrhea, he could promptly avail himself of resources in the community to restore his precoital state of health. Should not the pregnant woman's need to regain her prepregnant state of integrity be given equal consideration, or is equal justice more to be proclaimed than practiced?

Many variables are decisive to the determination of health. Forcing a woman to carry a pregnancy resentfully to term may not only be detrimental to her welfare but to her family's and the community's as well. The adverse consequences of maternal rejection have long been recognized as a major factor contributing to psychopathology. In a study done in Scandinavia,[52] researchers matched every child of an unmarried mother who applied for and was refused an abortion with the next "normal child" born in the same hospital. The investigation spanned twenty-one years. Children of women who were refused abortions were often picked up for antisocial or criminal behavior, received less education and more psychiatric treatment, and were more often exempt from military service because of physical defects. Human beings need to feel secure, to be loved, to belong, and to be accepted. In the absence of genuine human relationships within the family and the community, the mother who is spiritually, emotionally, and socially impoverished will be ill prepared to provide the child with the basic requisites for good health. Lacking access to abortion, she has also increased the likelihood of bringing into the world a child who, if not adoptable, nobody may really want. Indivisible from the former conclusions is the following ethical question: is it better to be born under conditions in which the essentials for enhancement of human existence are absent or not to be born at all? One must keep in mind, however, the fact that some individuals have found the strength to transcend inauspicious beginnings and to lead satisfying lives.

Conclusions

From conception to senescence the life process is one of becoming—self-actualization, or the fulfillment of potential. A basic supposition in considering self-actualization is that human beings do not have the right to maximize their potential at another's expense. Otherwise, personal autonomy in the pursuit of self-fulfillment, however ill defined or elusive, has always been a part of the American dream. The legal right to abortion for some, may symbolize a realization of that dream.

International Planned Parenthood Federation recently surveyed what amounts to 63% of the world's population for information relevant to family planning.[53] There was statistical indication that nearly one out of three pregnancies will be deliberately terminated. The reality of this projection is that more than one third of the women whom the maternity nurse encounters will be seeking abortion. Professional recognition and respect for this large, newly legal segment of the population warrants humanitarian consideration of their basic rights.

In historical perspective, no constitutionally guaranteed human right has yet been seen to retreat passively or permanently into the past. Although dissent may continue to flourish, the demand for legal abortion is not likely to cease. The nurse's right to believe that abortions are wrong is absolute, but basic to a democratic system of government is the recognition that freedom to believe should not limit the freedom of those who cannot conform or who are not bound by similar beliefs. Moreover, the precept of equal protection of rights under the law may be interpreted to include the right to control one's reproductive life. Just as one woman has the right to carry her pregnancy to term if she wishes, another has the right to terminate her pregnancy if unwanted. The woman who determinedly rejects her pregnancy and is forced to bear a child against her will cannot be forced to want or love the child. There may be a need to reflect more on the morality of compelling individuals to go against their consciences. To compel a woman to complete an unwanted and unwelcomed pregnancy may be as wrong as to compel a nurse who has conscientious objections to abortion to assist in one. Within the constraints of one's conscience, the issue of abortion should be faced as practically as possible.

Pragmatically the sensitive practitioner may be better able to protect new life through a commitment to programs that may prevent the need for abortion, such as education in family life and planning. The importance of working for social changes that make alternatives to abortion more acceptable cannot be overemphasized. Equal employment opportunities for the father and child care for the working mother, in addition to information about adoptive procedures, may help individuals to cope better with their economic and social circumstances. Certainly, increased humanism in present services will make people less hesitant to use them. Realistically the sensitive nurse also appreciates the fact that, because human beings have limitations, there are limits to human endurance and to the burdens that individuals can bear. Within the context of the times, nursing care to patients having discretionary abortions may be a vital component of human services.

Helpful to the patient contemplating a discretionary abortion is therapeutic communication. Cornish[54] states that unwanted pregnancy obliterates all other thoughts and concerns. In addition to exhibiting behaviors directly related to the dramatic changes in her body, the woman who does not desire to be pregnant may be in an acute state of tension and anxiety. She needs a great deal of emotional support to make a thoughtful and considered choice of abortion. She needs information about alternatives, to weigh them and their consequences, and to be certain that abortion is the soundest possible course of action available to her. She may need help in clarifying her own feelings and making sure that abortion is what *she* really wants and *not* simply what her boyfriend, husband, parents, or others recommend.

Anticipatory guidance is part of the nursing process: assessing the preabortion patient's need for knowledge and giving suitable explanations regarding procedures and preoperative and postoperative care are as significant for these patients as for any other surgical candidate. Preoperatively the patient should be allowed to disclose her fears—of pain, mutilation, sterility, death, or difficulties with future pregnancies and her doubts about having an abortion. Therapeutic communication can take place only in a nonthreatening atmosphere with people who sincerely want to help. Whatever information the patient needs should be given as objectively as possible, so that she can make a decision that is valid for her in her life situation. Having made a decision, she has the right to have it carried out under optimal circumstances, not the least of which is competent and compassionate implementation of the nursing process. In addition to other stressors, the patient may fear encountering contemptuous hostility from professionals who disagree with her abortion decision.[55]

Knowledgeable implementation of the nursing process involves using its predictive value and alerting the nurse to possible reactions to loss and the behavioral manifestations of grief. There may be more opportunity to help the patient cope with emotional trauma prior to than after an abortion because postabortal contact tends to be relatively brief.

The total experience of unwanted pregnancy and abortion may be associated with multiple losses—loss of a relationship with the putative father, loss of family regard and emotional and economic support, loss of social and self-esteem, and the loss of a part of oneself that held human potential. Although for "most women, abortion appears to be accompanied by few, if any, negative psychologic sequelae"[55] especially in the early months of pregnancy, continuity of care involves familiarizing the patient with community resources that may help in working out later conflicts of life problems, in addition to resources for contraceptive follow-up.

The woman who finds pregnancy untenable is in crisis, and crisis creates emotionally vulnerable individuals, who must be appreciated as such. Crisis intervention supports the human capacity for growth and change, to resolve problems, and to achieve a higher level of functioning. The nursing process may be helpful in reassuring the woman having an elective abortion that she is a worthy human being with the human right to make a mistake and to attempt to gain mastery over her life.

ETHICAL PROBLEM SOLVING

Because human beings generally seek regularity and uniformity, there is the rueful hope that change can occur without too much threat to one's personal sense of equanimity. However, ethical problem solving produces stress; principled thinking and creative growth in personal development are not devoid of pain, which is a consequence of the tension and anxiety engendered by uncertainty—one of the most distinctive features of a world that is not easily fathomed but must be faced.

Uncertainty may encourage ethical reflection, causing us to pause, to wonder, and to question the original premises of some of our beliefs. From such introspection we may find that some of our beliefs are dysfunctional in the kind of problem solving mandated by the tempo of our times. When we are uncertain, our mental energies are less likely to be developed to sustaining one idea; when our thoughts are guided along new lines, distance is placed between dogmatism and deliberation.

Ethical reflection can be a lonely companion for contemplation of the deep enigmas of life because there are no incontrovertible ethical truths waiting to be discovered either to confound or to comfort us. Whatever progress is made is on our own. One self-measure of progress may be increased ability to identify, and thus increased ability to handle, those behavioral responses that are nonfacilitating to therapeutic communication and thus to humanistic care.

Patient-care situations involving nurses in issues of life and death characterize the changing moral dilemmas indigenous to the beginning and at the end of the life continuum in the health care milieu. The need to concentrate on searching for ways to harmonize disparate ethical positions and to meet the human needs of patients are these dilemmas. Throughout life, caring, trust, empathy, sympathy, and respect are patterns of relatedness that support human uniqueness and dignity. Meaningful implementation of the nursing process requires that these humanistic approaches somehow cohere into responses that communicate a reverence for life and for the individual who must live it.

REFERENCES

1. American Nurses' Association Committee on Ethical, Legal and Professional Standards: Code for nurses with interpretive statements., Kansas City, Mo., 1976, The Association.
2. Silva, M.: Science, ethics, and nursing, American Journal of Nursing **74:**2004-2007, 1974.
3. Quinn, N., and Somers, A.: The Patient's Bill of Rights: a significant aspect of the consumer revolution, Nursing Outlook **22:**240-244, 1974.
4. Fagin, C.: Nurses' rights, American Journal of Nursing **75:**82-85, 1975.
5. American Hospital Association: A patient's bill of rights, Chicago, 1972, The Association.
6. Law and the courts, Modern Hospital **120:**33-34, 1973.
7. 1973 convention issues: proposed Resolution No. 1 on rights and responsibilities in nursing practice, Michigan Nurse Newsletter **46:**26, Sept., 1973.
8. Paulen, A.: Living with cancer: the rights of the patient and the rights of the nurse. In Peterson, B., and Kellogg, C., editors: Current practice in oncologic nursing, St. Louis, 1976, The C. V. Mosby Co., pp. 163-170.
9. The dying person's bill of rights, created at a workshop on the terminally ill patient and the helping person, held in Lansing, Michigan, American Journal of Nursing **75:**99, 1975.
10. Quint, J.: Obstacles to helping the dying, American Journal of Nursing **66:**1568-1571, 1966.
11. Beauchamp, B.: Euthanasia and the nurse practitioner, Nursing Forum **14:**58-59, 1975.
12. Halley, J., and Harvey, A.: Medical vs. legal definitions of death, Journal of the American Medical Association **204:**424-427, 1968.
13. Still, J.: The levels of life and semantic confusion, ETC: a review of general semantics **28:**9-21, March, 1971.
14. Sudnow, D.: Passing on, Englewood Cliffs, 1976, Prentice-Hall, Inc., p. 84.
15. Shindell, S.: The law in medical practice, Pittsburgh, 1966, University of Pittsburgh Press, p. 121.
16. Dedek, J.: Human life: some moral issues, New York, 1972, Sheed & Ward, Inc., p. 68.
17. Sanders, M., and Fisher, J.: The crisis in American medicine, New York, 1961, Harper & Row, Publishers, p. 135.
18. Ramsey, P.: Reference points in deciding about abortion. In Noonan, J., editor: The morality of abortions, Cambridge, Mass., 1972, Harvard University Press, pp. 94-97.
19. Dedek, op. cit., p. 125.
20. Ibid., p. 126.
21. Smith, D.: Some ethical considerations in caring for the dying, American Nurses' Association Clinical Sessions, New York, 1974, Appleton-Century-Crofts, p. 179.
22. Morrison, R.: Dying, Scientific American **229:**59-60, 1973.
23. Shindell, op. cit., p. 118.
24. Quint, J.: The nurse and the dying patient, New York, 1969, Macmillan, Inc., p. 98.
24a. Drakontides, A.: Drugs to treat pain, American Journal of Nursing **74:**508-513, 1974.
25. Murphy, T. M., Cancer pain, Postgraduate Medicine **53:**187-194, 1973.
26. Fletcher, J.: Ethics and euthanasia, American Journal of Nursing **73:**670-675, 1973.
27. Weber, L.: Ethics and euthanasia: another view, American Journal of Nursing **73:**1228-1231, 1973.
27a. Ibid., p. 1230.
28. Smith, H.: Ethics and new medicine, Nashville, Tenn., 1970, Abingdon Press, p. 166.
29. Goldstein, T.: Death and the law, The New York Times, p. 38, April 12, 1976.
30. Ramsey, op. cit., p. 100.
31. Foote, E.: The role of law (and lawyers) in medicine, Washington University Magazine **46:**28-29, Spring, 1976.
32. Hershey, N.: Students as staff nurses? American Journal of Nursing **67:**117, 1967.
33. Meyers, D.: The legal aspects of euthanasia, Bioscience, pp. 467-469, Aug., 1973.
34. Delsner, L.: High court bars giving a husband veto on abortion: parents also curbed, The New York Times, July 1, 1976, p. 1.
35. Lader, L.: Abortion II: making the revo-

lution, Boston, 1973, Beacon Press, p. 109.

36. Lanahan, C.: Anxieties and fears of patients seeking abortion. In McNall, L., & Galeener, J., editors: Current practice in obstetric and gynecologic nursing, St. Louis, 1976, The C. V. Mosby Co., p. 203.

37. Cornish, J.: Women's experiences with abortion. In McNall, L., and Galeener, J., editors: obstetric and gynecologic nursing, St. Louis, 1976, The C. V. Mosby Co., pp. 206-207.

38. De Beauvoir, S.: The second sex, translated by H. M. Parshley, New York, 1961, Alfred A. Knopf, Inc., p. 491.

39. Callahan, D.: Abortion: law, choice, and morality, New York, 1970, MacMillan, Inc., pp. 7-8.

40. Ibid, p. 8.

41. White, R.: Abortion and psychiatry. In Hall, R., editor: Abortion in a changing world, ed. 2, New York, 1968, Columbia University Press, p. 57.

42. Noonan, J.: An almost absolute value in history. In Noonan, J., editor: The morality of abortion, Cambridge, Mass., 1972, Harvard University Press, p. 57.

43. Dedek, op. cit., pp. 61-62.

44. Ramsey, op. cit., p. 73.

45. Stockhouse, M.: Abortion and anima-

tion. In Hall, R., editor: Abortion in a changing world, ed. 2., New York, 1968, Columbia University Press, p. 15.

46. Vaughn, P.: The pill turns twenty, New York Times Magazine, pp. 61-64, June 13, 1976.

47. Shainess, N.: Abortion and psychiatry. In Hall, R., editor: Abortion in a changing world, ed. 2, New York, 1968, Columbia University Press, p. 60.

48. Cornish, op. cit., p. 210.

49. Committee of psychiatry and law; The right to abortion: a psychiatric view, New York, 1970, Charles Scribner's Sons, p. 42.

50. Mecklenburg, F.: The indications for induced abortion. In Hilger, T., and Horan, D., editors: Abortion and social justice, New York, 1972, Sheed & Ward, Inc., p. 40.

51. Callahan, op. cit., pp. 132, 136.

52. LeRoux, R., Barnes, S., Gottesfeld, K., West, D., and Tolch, M.: Abortion, American Journal of Nursing **70**:1919-1925, 1970.

53. Cornish, op. cit., p. 205.

54. Ibid, p. 207.

55. Osofsky, H., and Osofsky, J.: The abortion experience: psychological and medical impact, New York, 1973, Harper & Row, Publishers, p. 10.

Decision making in communication—exercises in interpersonal relations

Part Two is presented in the form of fictionalized vignettes. Although drawn from real life, they are not exact replications of specific patient-care situations. They were made as realistic as possible to highlight some of the salient features of therapeutic communication. Because there is usually more than one communication principle operating in each exercise, the vignettes do not lend themselves to compartmental-ization within a chapter structure. The stories are presented in no special order, and the title of each suggests the content. There is a space left in front of each response so that the reader can make some notation of preference before comparing answer(s) with the discussion material that follows.

The response(s) preselected as correct is(are) italicized but with the clear recognition that the reader may decidedly disagree. The strength or weakness of words inheres in large measure in what the nurse's presence conveys. Since each reader brings much of herself to any situation, whether hypothetical or actual, this important variable could never be adequately taken into account in the individual presentations. How the nurse makes use of her presence may be of more significance than mere words; for just saying the "right" thing is no guarantee that the communication system will work smoothly and saying the "wrong" thing will not short-circuit the system forever. The effectiveness of verbal communication seems contingent on goodwill, and, although we cannot expect to make everyone feel better, communications that convey good-will seem to expand helping capacities. Knowing that the nurse is *for* and *with* them tends to provide the climate for patients to share what they are experiencing or feeling and offers solace as they bear what they feel. Thus the italicized response may well be an *oversimplification* and not at all consonant with the nurse's frame of reference or unique personal experiences in helping relationships.

Instead of reading Part Two of the book straight through, the reader may find more interest in returning to the vignettes from time to time. The disproportionate number dealing with the process of grief and dying may seem to indicate a morbid preoccupation, but the intent is to reflect professional concern to better help individuals as they live these experiences.

THE PATIENT WHO LOSES A BODY PART

Danny Southerland, 31 years of age, is well known locally as a folksinger. He appears frequently on radio and television talk shows and projects a personable, confident image. Lately he has been having a throbbing pain behind his right eye but put off seeing his ophthalmologist, Dr. Bender, until the pain became unbearable. Examination revealed that a tumor was causing his symptoms, and Mr. Southerland was admitted to the hospital that same evening. The physician informed him that there was no way of telling whether the tumor was benign or malignant until a sample of cells could be examined by the pathologist at the time of surgery, and, if the cells were malignant, the eye would have to be sacrificed as a lifesaving measure. Miss Drayton, the day nurse, had her first contact with Mr. Southerland when she administered his preoperative medication. Dr. Bender was in the room starting an infusion and explaining to the patient that, although the operation might turn out to be a simple one, a general anesthetic would have to be given. Mr. Southerland's only comment was that he would be glad when the operation was all over and the excruciating pain was gone. During surgery, pathologic study showed the tumor to be a form of melanoma, and the patient's right eye was enucleated. When Mr. Southerland is returned to the ward, Nurse Drayton reads the surgical notes, picks up the postoperative orders, and goes to check his vital signs. As she is applying the blood pressure cuff, the patient suddenly grips her arm and says, "Please I must know. Did the doctor have to remove my eye?"

Which response by Nurse Drayton probably shows the soundest professional judgment?

_____ 1. "I am truly sorry, but the laboratory report was not favorable. The tumor and all the surrounding tissue had to be removed to save your life."

_____ 2. "I can understand why you seem so anxious, but I do not know with any degree of certainty the extent of the operative procedure. However, I am sure that Dr. Bender did everything possible to ensure a favorable outcome."

_____ 3. "I can see that you are worried, but I cannot answer any questions about your surgery without first speaking to your doctor. If you like, I'll find out if he is available to see you now."

_____ 4. "From the kind of bandage you have and the length of time that you were in the operating room, there is the possibility that you had a serious problem."

Discussion

1. Is based on two assumptions: the patient's right to know and his capability to assimilate information rationally, independent of the circumstances. It is the doctor's prerogative to inform the patient of his diagnosis. Whether or not he does so, for the nurse to get his views on the matter is always ethical as well as judicious. The patient's right to have his questions answered openly and honestly does not impose an obligation to be fulfilled without an assessment of his readiness to know. Considerable personal knowledge regarding Mr. Southerland's feelings about his body, his level of emotional maturity, his coping mechanisms, and the probable impact of the loss on his life-style is needed. Until all these variables have been carefully weighed, one needs to be prudent in communicating to the patient the fact of cancer. We know that Mr. Southerland has had little time to adjust to an impending loss and change in body image. We also know that the eye and the ego are symbolically inseparable. Moreover, people do not invade each other's personal space without strong motivation. Patients tend to grip a nurse's arm when they are in pain or panic, which can follow the threat of or actual loss of something highly valued. Grief follows such losses, and behavior in the initial stages of shock and disbelief is highly individualistic. The premise that the sooner the grieving process is initiated the better is based on due consideration of the patient's physical, psychologic, and social well-being. The behavior of a postoperative patient not fully recovered from anesthesia may be unpredictable at best. A reasoned choice to share with such a patient information that could precipitate a severe emotional reaction must carry with it a willingness to accept responsibility for the consequences.

2. Is unlikely to build a reservoir of goodwill, on which effective implementation of the nursing process depends. The patient's anxiety will probably increase if the first professional that he relates to in the ward is uninformed about matters directly relating to his care, comfort, and perhaps even his life. Should he perceive a discrepancy between the nurse's verbal and nonverbal behavior, he may resist the physical, as well as psychologic proximity on which his recovery and eventual adjustment may depend. Mr. Southerland's nonverbal cues are indications of the extent of his insecurity and difficulty in maintaining self-control, due to fear. Crucial to a patient's sense of safety is the development of trust and confidence in the staff. This

is one reason why dishonesty and false reassurance are rarely if ever satisfactory options.

3. Seems most indicative of sound professional judgment. It lets the patient know that the nurse is not withholding information deliberately but simply does not now have the authority to divulge medical data. Some may consider this "passing the buck" and avoiding the issue. It is. However, the preexisting relationship between the physician and patient, as well as the physician's right to discuss diagnosis in the manner that he believes to be in the best interest of his patient, must be respected. Without prior consultation the nurse has no way of knowing whether Dr. Bender has selected someone from the patient's social network to be present to support the patient when he learns that he had/has a cancerous condition. Unless the nurse knows much more about the patient and has permission to disclose his diagnosis, the physician whom Mr. Southerland trusts and has confidence in, would seem to be the most capable person to judge how much information the patient can tolerate or accept.

4. Is an example of parrying—sometimes useful in gaining time to assess the patient's reaction to the intrusion of reality in small stages. However, the nurse needs to be aware of the fact that this approach may exacerbate, rather than allay, anxiety and provide a stimulus for more specific questions by the patient. Selective and appropriately timed information given in this situation would seem to require the collaborative efforts of the physician and nurse. Should Mr. Southerland respond to the nurse's communication by asking, "How serious a problem?" a tactful or satisfactory answer that does not divulge his diagnosis would be extremely difficult to find.

TEACHING NUTRITION

You are a nurse in a metabolic clinic. Regina Allen, a 25-year-old clerk-typist, is being treated for Graves' disease—a condition characterized by overactivity of the thyroid gland, with acceleration in the rate of all the bodily processes. The patient's chief complaints are weakness, fatigue, and weight loss, even though she eats an enormous amount of food. In addition to antithyroid medications, her physician has prescribed a high-calorie diet to provide for Miss Allen's increased energy needs, to prevent further weight loss, and to replace that already lost. The doctor has requested you to review with the patient her therapeutic regimen with special emphasis on nutritional guidance.

Which *initial* approach would probably be the most helpful in assessing the kinds of nutritional information that the patient needs?

_____ 1. "Miss Allen, try to remember, if you can, everything you ate and drank yesterday."

_____ 2. "Miss Allen, here are pictures of the basic four food groups. Please point out those foods you usually include in your diet."

_____ 3. "Miss Allen, can you tell me what you usually have for breakfast, lunch, dinner, and snacks?"

_____ 4. "When you last went grocery shopping, Miss Allen, what kinds of food did you buy?"

Discussion

1. Would probably be the best mode of inquiry initially because it most closely adheres to a basic axiom of interviewing—begin where the patient is. Information should be requested in a clear, concise, and unbiased manner to facilitate spontaneous responses. Although there are a number of sophisticated tools for obtaining data about food habits of patients, one means suggested by Williams* for use with clinic patients is asking the patient to recall every item of food or nutrient taken during the preceding 24 hours. This approach, combined with other communication techniques, such as listening and encouragement, may stimulate disclosure of details of Miss Allen's daily eating pattern in a fairly valid manner. Once a general idea of her nutritional intake is obtained in a nonthreatening manner, the nurse may want to explore more specifically with Miss Allen the approximate amount of each food, its method of preparation, the times of day that it is consumed, and similar data necessary for developing with the patient a personalized and therapeutic diet pattern. In essence, the patient is given more leeway in relating her dietary history and telling her story in her own way as it comes to her. This may give a better picture of the patient's established preferences, which any diet modification and sample menu planning should be built.

2. Would be a means of stimulating recollection only if the foods listed on the "basic four" charts are indigenous to Miss Allen's life-style or her cultural background. If not, this approach may communicate to the patient the false premise that foods predominant in the American culture are the most nutritious and desirable. If the patient's responses are rigidly structured, she may hesitate to communicate information pertinent to mutual identification of her true dietary needs. Once the nurse knows what kinds of food the patient eats, she may want to use this information to check against the nutrient groups to see if the patient's diet is well balanced and where caloric additions are needed. However, visual aids that suggest responses may also affect validity.

_____
*Williams, S. R.: Essentials of nutrition and diet therapy, St. Louis, 1974, The C. V. Mosby Co., p.133.

3. May reduce the level of patient participation by communicating the expectation that the patient's eating habits are *routinized* into a standard, set pattern. If the patient experiences strong feelings of status and value differences between herself and the nurse, she may give invalid responses to guard against making disclosures that might disparage her in some way; for example, instead of saying that she omits breakfast routinely or eats dinner leftovers in the morning, Miss Allen may try to save face by giving the all-American breakfast fare of bacon, eggs, juice, coffee, and toast. Then, too, if the patient eats continuously all day, she may forget to mention or to place the foods under the preselected categories. Just as there are differences in other forms of human behavior, there are differences in eating habits, and the patient should be permitted to approach the topic in ways that facilitate making her uniqueness known.
4. Would seem to put undue pressure on the patient to recall details of an event that, even if recent, might offer little relevant information concerning her daily eating habits, since she might purchase few groceries simply because she eats out often or a large amount of foods of which some are favored only by her guests. Certainly information about the patient's likes and dislikes, as well as the amount of money budgeted for food, will be helpful to the nurse but might be a logical by-product of the first response, which would seem to get to the heart of the matter somewhat more quickly.

FEE SETTING AND THE VISITING NURSE

Miss Laine, a 69-year-old diabetic, was referred to the visiting nurse service for health supervision after hospitalization for an acute episode of elevated blood sugar. Specifically the hospital requested a continuation of health care planned to prevent extreme manifestations of diabetes and to help the patient conserve her capacities for independent functioning. Nurse Alvarez called Miss Laine to discuss referral and reasons for the visit and to plan a date. In making the home visit, Nurse Alvarez found the patient to be spry, mentally alert, and self-sufficient, although living alone in a small, cheerless apartment in what was once a luxury hotel. The patient stated that as a former governess she is ineligible for social security benefits and lives off her savings, which have been supplemented over the years by occasional monetary gifts from children of her former employers. Having no prepaid health care plan to defray expenses of hospitalization, the patient reported that a large part of her savings had been spent for this purpose.

Further discussion disclosed that Miss Laine had little to do with the other tenants in the building, who were mostly elderly like herself—transient or indigent. However, she did manage to attend church almost every Sunday. For several years her diabetes was supervised by a private physician. Her condition could be controlled by diet alone, and she decided to decrease the frequency of her visits because she never had "serious problems." Two events seem definitely related to the patient's economic status: the cost of visits to the doctor was a factor in her decision to use his services rarely, and she was including many more carbohydrates than appropriate in her diet because the cost of other kinds of food that she preferred was often prohibitive. When Nurse Alvarez mentioned the possibility of obtaining food stamps, Miss Laine indignantly replied that she wanted "no contact whatsoever with the welfare center" that administered the program. Although the patient was reluctant to give an exact budgetary breakdown, she strongly intimated that after paying $145 per month for rent and utilities, she had "barely enough to get by."

There was mutual agreement that the priority of care at this time was proper menu planning, since this would best sustain the medical gains made during her period of hospitalization. Visits were jointly planned for three times a week at first, to be more widely spaced when less direct assistance was needed to help the patient maintain her capacity to care for herself. At the conclusion of this exchange a booklet containing such information as explanations of nursing, how to contact the agency, and a suggested fee schedule was reviewed with Miss Laine. The nurse explained that, although the listed full fee per visit was $22.75, this could be adjusted in accordance with the particular patient's economic circumstances. After reading over the fee schedule, Miss Laine reached into her sweater pocket, retrieved two quarters, and without looking up deposited the money on a table within the nurse's reach.

Which approach by the nurse would probably *best* maintain the rapport established with the patient thus far?

_____ 1. Informing Miss Laine that if the fee adds to her economic burdens payment will be waived.
_____ 2. Suggesting to Miss Laine that perhaps she would prefer to wait and make a contribution to the agency when she has more funds.
_____ 3. Thanking Miss Laine, making out a receipt for the fee, and handing the receipt to her, without further discussion.
_____ 4. Suggesting to Miss Laine that she would have much less hardship if she applied for Medicaid, which also helps cover the cost of nursing services.

Discussion

1. May tell the patient in so many words that the thought processes she used to make a decision were exercises in futility. First, she is granted freedom of choice in the fee payment; then her competency is questioned. There was sufficient preliminary discussion to allow the patient to set her own fee; after she has done so, the proffered payment should be accepted. Her avoidance of eye contact with the nurse and the manner in which she offered the coins suggest uncer-

tainty that the amount will be found satisfactory. More important than the intrinsic worth of the 50 cents may be an intense need to preserve feelings of self-worth by disassociating herself from charity. This conclusion is especially significant if the patient was reared in a social climate in which allegiance to the value of self-reliance makes her resist affiliation with anything vaguely suggesting a dole. Waiving the fee may inadvertently seem to delegate the patient to an inferior status, reinforcing a dependency role that she does not want. Such a role tends to counter feelings of personal autonomy. Should the patient perceive herself as being placed in an unfavorable light, she may resist and withdraw from a relationship in which such a devastating blow has been dealt to her pride. Miss Laine must be made to feel that what she can afford to pay is just as significant as a full fee. This would be in keeping with her well-defined social value of "earning her keep."

2. Seemingly gives the patient the opportunity to withdraw her offer gracefully. However, suggesting an alternative method of payment when the patient has already selected one may have the humiliating side effect of implying that the first offer was inadequate and that she should wait until she can pay more. Miss Laine may well misinterpret the offer to defer payment as an effort to capitalize on the fact that she sometimes receives gifts of money. Patients need to feel that they are full participants in a therapeutic relationship from the start. Payment of a fee may be considered therapeutic because individuals tend to feel freer to express dissatisfaction with a service that they pay for, as well as to show more inclination to relinquish one that is no longer needed. Moreover, because they see that they have a concrete, vested interest in the relationship, they tend better to maximize opportunities to plan and implement their care. If the patient wishes to pay for services rendered the payment should not be deferred. Fee payment is an expression of faith in the contract made with the nurse, as well as acknowledgment of nursing service as a valuable component of health care.

3. Would seem to maintain rapport best because it demonstrates awareness that nursing intervention that supports human strivings for independence and self-esteem is essential to successful restoration and maintenance of health. The greater the patient's confidence in herself and the stronger her desire to maintain herself in her home environment, the more receptive she may be to modifying or adjusting those aspects of her life that pose threats to health care goals. Hospitalization imposes reliance on others to fulfill one's basic needs. This dependency, coupled with a realistic confrontation with waning physical powers, may initiate a cycle of diminished self-regard and self-assertiveness that should be interrupted. One means of doing

so is to foster in the patient the belief that she is a full card-carrying partner in her therapeutic regimen and not just a passive recipient of care. Axiomatically this society finds creditable the assumption that one does not get "something for nothing." In other words, whatever one receives without effort may be considered valueless. Although there are no clear-cut norms for this kind of patient-care situation, one might reasonably conclude that fees seem to reaffirm the worth of a given service and that the ministrations of the nurse are more likely to be beneficial when they are perceived as being worthwhile. Admittedly there is a risk that Miss Laine may be paying more than her budget permits. Fee schedules, like all phases of nursing service, necessitate constant reassessment. They are not irrevocable. Delegating a patient to a nonpaying position, which she may presently feel to be beneath her dignity, may be more harmful.

4. Is more representative of a long-range than an immediate goal. For those unfamiliar with Medicaid, let me explain that it is a prepaid health care plan under the auspices of city or state social service, usually meaning welfare agencies. However, the key to eliminating this answer is the patient's demonstrated desire to reserve information about her exact financial status. More time is needed to establish a trusting relationship before she will feel comfortable in discussing her qualifications for assistance. Currently she seems concerned about being treated as a "poor" patient and unreceptive to the idea that a taxpayer has a right to reimbursement in the form of social services.

A CHILD WITH ACUTE LYMPHOBLASTIC LEUKEMIA

Timothy, 3½ years of age, was readmitted to the pediatric unit 4 days ago for treatment of the advanced stages of lymphoblastic leukemia. His illness was first diagnosed when he was nearing his third birthday. The sequential use of a combination of prednisone and vincristine could not prevent the pathologic cells from infiltrating his central nervous system. He is a middle child, with an 18-month-old sister and an 8 year-old brother. His mother visits him during the day and his father in the evenings after work. The medical reports that the family receives are not good. Timothy, now subject to headaches, nausea and vomiting, fatigue, and joint pain, is dying. One day after an episode of vomiting, as Nurse Lehman is cleaning him up, Timothy angrily exclaims, "I wish you would drop dead!"

Which of the following interpretations of Timothy's statement to Nurse Lehman would probably be the most insightful?

_____ 1. Timothy feels abandoned and is displacing the anger that he feels toward his mother to the nurse, a maternal surrogate.

_____ 2. Timothy's death wish for Nurse Lehman is a manifestation of concern with the idea of his own death.

_____ 3. Timothy does not wish to be disturbed and would like the nurse to go away and leave him alone.

_____ 4. Timothy is frightened and wants the nurse to hold him close and stop giving him care for a while.

Discussion

1. Does not seem to be the best interpretation of Timothy's message. Certainly the 3 year-old child responds to separation from the mother or any person who fulfills this role with total and absolute outrage, and a valid conclusion would be that a child who did not feel secure enough to vent fury directly on the mother might displace such feelings. However, Timothy's very existence is dependent on his mother who feeds, clothes, puts him to bed, makes decisions, and gives directions. Mother means everything—understanding and security. Therefore Timothy is much too dependent, or reliant, on mothering to harbor either conscious or unconscious wishes to banish her. He could not risk losing what is so badly needed and central to a child at his maturation level—a mother's presence.

2. Is also incorrect. To a 3-year-old child death has no personal meaning, and Timothy is not aware that his individual existence is coming to an end. This is because he sees himself and his parents as a unified whole. Since he does not yet conceive of himself as a separate being, he does not have to worry about the possiblity of nonbeing. However, in the process of dying he may react sensitively to the feelings and activities around him: if his parents are fearful, he will be fearful; if the staff is despondent, he will be despondent. He may have learned to associate the staff with unpleasant experiences. People with strange faces do unpredictable things. Sometimes they come to comfort and at other times to hurt him with needles for medications and blood transfusions. He responds to the pain of bodily deterioration with the strength of a $3\frac{1}{2}$-year-old child—with cries of distress, bewilderment, anger, and frustration. He knows that he is somehow being threatened but believes that no permanent harm can come to him because his parents live.

3. Would seem to be the best interpretation of Timothy's message. To Timothy, death is only a temporary disappearance, a process of coming and going. Whatever change occurs in a relationship is only for the time being, and the original status is certain to be restored. In Timothy's world, things do not just happen; one's thoughts can cause them to happen. Thus, with the reasoning of a child, Timothy believes that, if he wishes hard enough, Nurse Lehman will simply go away for a while and leave him alone. Since absences last only a short time, the nurse cannot go too far away. Hence she could quickly return if summoned.

4. Does not show the best understanding of a 3 year-old toddler's primitive ideas about death. To a child of this tender age, death and
temporary absence are the same. Timothy probably thinks that he
is being mistreated, since, in the final stages of his illness even the
most gentle care may increase his discomfort. To Timothy, everything
is black or white—good or bad. Bad people hurt you; because Nurse
Lehman is bad at the moment, she needs to be banished.

THE DEMANDING PATIENT—Part I

Mrs. Hexter, 72 years of age, was admitted to a nursing home after an
extended period of hospitalization for a fracture of her left hip. Because of
the aftereffects of a stroke suffered over a year previously, the patient lived
with her son, his wife, and their two children. Mrs. Hexter was widowed at
an early age and likes to talk about how she almost single-handedly helped
her son to achieve the status of engineer. The patient attributes her present
injury to a fall in the bathtub as she attempted to climb out unaided while
her daughter-in-law was gossiping on the phone. Although now ambulatory
with the use of a walker, the patient was placed in the nursing home because
the family could not cope with continuity of her care. Mrs. Hexter apparently
accepted their plan stoically until it became an actuality. From the moment
of admission she barraged the staff with a litany of complaints: her room
did not have a picturesque view, and her roommate was hard of hearing;
she wanted to use the bedpan rather than get up to go to the bathroom
if she were lying down; she demanded to be first for everything—morning
care, breakfast, and bed making—yet she complained to her physician that
the staff would not let her sleep. For a while, she refused all medications
because a prescribed tranquilizer had left her extremely lethargic and "doped
up." The doctor states that the patient, although demanding, is not disoriented
and admits that caring for her is indeed difficult. Mrs. Hexter refuses to assist
with her hygienic care and, when requested to do so, angrily retorts, "That's
what my son is paying you good money for!" When she is in a particularly
irascible mood, she declines all care and then points out her disheveled
appearance to everyone as proof that she is neglected. Although Mrs. Hexter
is indiscriminate in her tongue-lashing, her special target is Nurse Dowd, who
is primarily responsible for planning and implementing the patient's care. When
this nurse brought the patient's medications to her one evening, Mrs. Hexter,
after summarizing her grievances for the day, became strangely quiet and
compliant. Then as the nurse was leaving the bedside, the patient remarked,
"You always seem to be in a hurry; now, you don't like me much, do you?"

What understanding of the situation should Nurse Dowd strive to
communicate to the patient at this opportune moment?

_____ 1. "I cannot always do exactly what you want, but this does not
mean that I dislike or deliberately avoid you. However, I must

admit that we could help you better if you didn't continually try to frustrate our efforts."

____ 2. "All the stress of adjusting to this new situation must make you feel uncared for sometimes. I'll try to find more time to familiarize you with the daily routines; then you will not feel so lonely and neglected."

____ 3. "Well, since you are in such a good mood and seem able to take a joke, quite honestly you wouldn't exactly be my nominee for a Mrs. Congeniality award!"

____ 4. "Well, since you asked for it, the truth of the matter is that I often feel downright discouraged and upset with both myself and you because, frankly, whatever I do, it never seems to be what you need."

Discussion

1. Communicates a superficial concern for the patient's feelings and then goes on to inform Mrs. Hexter that her personal conduct does not follow the rules of propriety for the sick role, that is to cooperate and comply preferably in a cheerful manner. Implicit in this response is the division of the interpersonal relationship into "good and bad guy" roles. Although health care providers are working diligently on the patient's behalf, Mrs. Hexter, instead of being appreciative, displays a recalcitrance that makes their role more difficult; although staff members do not go out of their way to avoid her, their ministrations would be more beneficial if she would just be gracious enough to accept the norms of the sick role. This reply shows a negative regard for her efforts to retain a unique identity; hence it is not constructive in helping her to give up her self-defeating behavior. More likely, in protest of this bad guy image and protection of an already traumatized ego, Mrs. Hexter will persist in her stereotypic, alienating behavior.

2. Conveys to the patient that, although the reasons for her intransigence are understood, nevertheless they do not have to be dealt with because the obvious remedy is to accelerate the process of socialization to the sick role. Mrs. Hexter's deviant behavior is met with an air of noblesse oblige; the patient's difficulties can be readily resolved once she becomes more accustomed to regularity. In the first two responses, no attempt is made to use the patient's communications as an opportunity to examine and expand the relationship in a more mutually satisfying manner. The onus is on Mrs. Hexter to change her identity —to change herself—if she is ever to achieve a state of equilibrium.

3. May also be considered an unsatisfactory response to Mrs. Hexter's efforts to initiate conversation on a deep level of personal meaning.

The nurse either fails to take seriously the patient's behavioral clues or chooses to misinterpret them to avoid responding other than superficially to the deep undercurrents of feeling. Although humor can be an excellent medium for bringing people together, it may also be a means of avoiding an experience that threatens to be painful. This maneuver may cause the patient to feel inadequate at or incapable of getting through to people to achieve relationships of human concern and involvement. Moreover, the nurse may have missed an opportunity to pursue the patient's observations with an openness that could be a positive turning point in the patient-care situation.

4. Seems to be a genuine human response to a difficult situation and may clear the air for mutual participation in seeking solutions to the problem. The patient has revealed her perceptions of the situation. The possibility that one is disliked is painful to contemplate, much less give voice to. Even though honest feedback and validation of her observations may be upsetting to both patient and nurse, Mrs. Hexter is entitled to this approach, which seems essential if behavioral changes are to be based on accurate data, rather than distorted environmental cues and fantasy. If Nurse Dowd has persistent feelings of discomfort in the situation and attempts to act otherwise, the patient will sense the discrepancy and discontinue efforts to disclose her feelings about herself and her changed life situation. Aiken and Aiken have stated that "the demanding or difficult patients provide an excellent example of inappropriate niceness."* Instead of facing the situation directly, the nurse may smilingly avoid the patient and provide him with no clues as to why he is being rejected. In facilitating genuineness, the nurse neither burdens the patient with her feelings nor attacks him but *shares* those feelings relevant to working toward a therapeutic relationship. By revealing her own authentic feelings, the nurse may provide a role model that permits and encourages the patient to do likewise. Saupe† concludes that patients denied an opportunity to discover the real feelings of others are handicapped in interpersonal relationships; when the patient is trusted with uncontrived emotions, whether positive or negative, he can respond more appropriately, begin to feel like a true participant in the relationship, and assume his *fair* share of responsibility for resolving interpersonal conflict. Genuineness, instead of being harmful, can strengthen feelings of self-worth in both nurse and patient, and this positive sense of identity can provide a valuable beginning for a productive, truly human encounter.

---

*From Aiken, L., and Aiken, J.: A systematic approach to the evaluation of interpersonal relationships, American Journal of Nursing **73:**863-867, 1973.
†Saupe, P.: How do you feel, nurse? American Journal of Nursing **74:**1105, 1974.

THE DEMANDING PATIENT—Part II

In spite of the staff's attempts to anticipate Mrs. Hexter's identifiable needs, respond to her reasonable requests promptly and allow her to make decisions concerning her care whenever possible, as well as spend more time with her, the patient's behavior, although modified, continues unabated. She demonstrates a remarkable resilience of spirit in resisting distractions from her campaign to control her life in her own way. She refuses to participate in any occupational or recreational therapy and mingles with other patients seemingly only long enough to add their complaints to her own list for personal delivery to Nurse Dowd. Staff members have concluded that the patient's modus operandi may be her level of optimal functioning and are actually becoming fond of her. The Christmas season is approaching; her family, who visit frequently, will be spending the holidays out of town with her daughter-in-law's relatives. Today, after a rather brief recital of wrongs, Mrs. Hexter, sighing deeply, concludes, "We are just a bunch of useless old people put out to pasture. What did we do to deserve this?"

Which response by Nurse Dowd would probably show the *most* empathetic understanding of the patient's comments?

_____ 1. "I suspect that you are speaking for yourself. You seem to feel that you are being punished and that perhaps you have done something wrong."

_____ 2. "I think you are telling me as much about yourself as you are about patients in general. Being in a position of having to be helped must be depressing to you after taking care of yourself for so many years."

_____ 3. "Holidays can be depressing when you are away from family and friends. I have felt the same way sometimes but found that if I keep busy the whole picture pretty much changes."

_____ 4. "Even though there have been major changes in most patients' lives, this does not mean that life can't be fulfilling. Since you are able to speak up so well for the group, what do you think should be done?"

Discussion

1. Recognizes that perhaps the patient's message has a self-referent meaning but shows little empathy because the rhetorical question that usually imparts more emotions rather than asks for information is responded to with probing. Rhetorical questions are pseudoquestions used to give an air of neutrality and objectivity to the expression of strong feelings that one is not ready to "own." Interpretation of such feelings as having an underlying assumptive base of guilt and fear of retribution may create so much tension and anxiety in Mrs. Hexter at this time as to aggravate her state of disequilibrium.

Consideration should be given to the possibility that the patient is conveying deep feelings of hopelessness and helplessness. As to what she did to deserve this, the only humane response, if the nurse thinks that she knows enough to answer, is "nothing." This answer, then, adds more to the patient's remarks than she is likely to be able to use constructively in her present state.

2. Seems to show the most empathetic understanding of Mrs. Hexter's remarks. Knowledge of the patient's background, in addition to her present life circumstances and communication, would seem to justify the conclusion that the patient was in a state of despondency. Furthermore, the second response is a reflection of what is known; although this is not necessarily a precondition for empathy, it may facilitate a more accurate perception of the patient's troubled world. The second reply also best assesses and reflects the feeling tone of the communication; that is, the nurse understands what it may be like to see one's powers of self-determination and autonomy on the wane. Empathy is an enabling technique. If the patient feels understood, she is more likely to move to deeper levels of exploration of feelings.

3. Nurse Dowd tries to explain the patient's feelings away in accordance with the nurse's preconceived frame of reference. Her observation concerning festive events and depression may be accurate, but she does not allow time for the patient's personal reflections about the significance of the holiday or exploration of painful feelings associated with the event. Instead, the nurse's probably meaningless suggestions about how to cope will more than likely cut off two-way conversation. Instead of showing concern for the patient, this response, in effect, is meant to control her behavior.

4. Would probably be the least empathetic response because it demonstrates a kind of intellectualizing that fails to synchronize the patient's emotional state with her verbal message. Instead of finding someone to share her sorrow, the patient is urged to give up her despondent egocentricity and to problem solve for the group. Often individuals speak in generalizations to soften hurt. Furthermore, the patient needs her potential strengths channeled into helping her overcome her distress, instead of being redirected on behalf of the group. By responding to the literal content of Mrs. Hexter's message, Nurse Dowd initiates a discussion by which she avoids responding to the patient's feelings.

A VICTIM OF RAPE

Linda McNeil, a 19-year-old college student, was allegedly raped while returning to the dormitory alone after attending a late movie. She is brought to the hospital by her roommate, Gail, and two policemen. Nurse Ford has arranged for the group to converse in a private room while awaiting the arrival of Dr. Pinckney, the gynecologist on duty. Miss McNeil responds to the officers in monosyllables, interspersed with long periods of silence, and gives a rather incoherent, disconnected picture of the recent events. The policemen ask to speak with Nurse Ford alone; after a brief conference the decision is made that she should be left alone with Linda and Gail for a while to try to ease the patient's anxiety.

Which communication by Nurse Ford would probably make the *best* use of this time?

_____ 1. "You seem to have had as much as you can take, Miss McNeil. However, the policemen don't mean to upset you. It is legally important for you to answer their questions as completely as possible when they return. You may even feel better once that is done."

_____ 2. "Miss McNeil, Dr. Pinckney will be here shortly. Although you seem exhausted, he must examine you and make some necessary tests. Perhaps using this time to discuss what has to be done and why will make it a little easier for you."

_____ 3. "I know that you've been through a harrowing ordeal and are upset. It may help if you can tell Gail and me exactly what you are feeling right now."

_____ 4. "I know it hurts to talk about it, and I wish there were a better way. Please let Gail and me help you sort out the facts while they are still fresh in your mind, and we will relay the information to the officers and doctor for you."

Discussion

1. May be more beneficial to the police officers than to the patient. No approach with an implicit demand is appropriate at this time, since the patient has already been subjected to an experience lacking the element of consent. Communications of a sensitive nature are extremely stressful and become even more so when they are structured. Linda needs to be permitted to recall the circumstances of the alleged assault in her own way and to express herself as her thoughts come to her, no matter how disorganized they may be. Getting a concise picture of what happened may take a great deal of time, but the patient should be supported on her own terms, even though this does not make the task of the policemen easier.

2. Does not take into consideration the possibility that Linda is nonverbally communicating the fact that she feels psychologically insecure. Because she is having difficulty in talking about a past assault on her person, this may not be the opportune moment to prepare for

what may well represent another one. To put oneself in the patient's place is to see that pelvic examinations involve a disarray of clothing and forced human contact with an authority figure. Symbolically, such procedures may reproduce the rape experience and reinforce feelings of trauma that the patient presently seems unable to face. A suitable explanation concerning medical intervention may be necessary but this is not the priority of the moment. Procedures can be explained as they are carried out.

3. Would probably have the greatest therapeutic impact in the available span of time. This is because of the attempt to communicate to the patient that details surrounding the incident are insignificant compared to the meaning of the experience for her. Recounting facts involves the concious self, but expressions of feelings mobilize the total self; hence they are more valid indicators of the hurt that the patient is living through. This interaction is likely to create a supportive atmosphere that communicating to Linda that the nurse has no objective but to share and try to alleviate some of the hurt. When feelings of fear, anger, and frustration decrease in intensity, the patient may be better able to recall the data requested. More importantly, however, acceptance of the patient now and sympathetic encouragement in the expression of feelings seem to follow principles basic to the prevention of permanent psychologic impairment.

4. Acknowledges Linda's feeling tone but again suggests that she should follow someone else's lead. The implication in this interaction is that systemized data gathering is more important than the person whom the data directly concern. The nurse may be well intentioned; nonetheless, she is engaging in a subtle form of interrogation. Aside from the fact that the policemen and the physician may desire a firsthand account, the paramount task of the nurse at this time is to communicate to the patient that she has a professional ally and companion in her pain.

THE PATIENT WITH A VENEREAL DISEASE—Part I

Mrs. Miriam Bennett is a 24-year-old attractive and vivacious waitress who works in a busy delicatessen across the street from Dr. Elting's office. One day on her lunch hour, she came to the office seeking treatment for a small painless ulceration on her lower lip. She stated that, although she has been partially disguising the lesion with makeup for more than a week, she was self-conscious about the blemish and found it an unaesthetic distraction in her line of work. Mrs. Bennett seemed to believe that, because she handles glasses, dishes, and silverware used by customers, she might have picked up some type of infection in this manner. After taking her history, examining the lesion, and getting a smear for a dark-field microscopic study, Dr. Elting drew a blood sample and requested that she return 3 days later. On keeping her appointment, Mrs. Bennett was informed by the physician that the ulcer on her lip is a chancre caused by syphilis and that her husband also needed to be examined. The doctor asked Nurse Harrison to give the patient benzathine penicillin G, 2.4 million units intramuscularly, and also a follow-up appointment. When alone with the nurse, Mrs. Bennett tearfully stated, "I've been married for over five years to David, and I have never even looked at another man. How could he do such a thing to me? I don't think I can even look him in the face to discuss it!"

Which response by Nurse Harrison would probably show the best understanding of the situation?

_____ 1. "I can see that this is a shock to you. It may ease your mind to know that the prescribed injection will cure your condition. The important thing is to take care of yourself and your immediate problem by beginning the treatment as you have done."

_____ 2. "In any intense relationship, individuals do things sometimes that make us hate as well as love them, and you have every reason to feel as strongly as you do."

_____ 3. "Fidelity in marriage seems to be important to you. It must really hurt inside to feel betrayed by someone whom you trust."

_____ 4. "Although it may be hard for you, your husband must be told right away so that he can be treated. Avoiding discussion of the problem will only make it more difficult to resolve. A referral for joint marital counseling may also be useful at this time."

Discussion

1. Is meant to be reassuring, but facts about Mrs. Bennett's physical status may fall on deaf ears because the patient has shifted her psychic energies from concern with symptoms to concern with self. Her verbalizations of indignation and bewilderment may be the consequence of a staggering blow to her self-image. Mrs. Bennett's needs are not exactly informational at this particular time. The interpersonal relationship with her husband is now also the focus of some of her anxieties.

2. Reflects an intensity of emotion that the patient's message does not convey. We do not know how Mrs. Bennett feels about her husband, although we can surmise that it is more than indifference. In the second response, Nurse Harrison seems to be identifying with the wife and aligning herself against the husband. Then, too, there is the subtle suggestion that hatred is an expected response to deep hurt—to infidelity. Even if the patient expressed outright hostility toward her husband, one would listen but be careful not to pass judgment in any way on the husband's behavior.

3. Probably shows the best understanding of Mrs. Bennett's situation because it seems to fit best the feelings sifted from the flood of responses. When Nurse Harrison reflects the feelings in Mrs. Bennett's statements back to her, this may communicate to the patient that the experience from her point of view is understood. When feelings concerning a problem are brought out into the open and anxiety is decreased, the problem itself may be put into better perspective, and the patient may be able to start thinking constructively about her situation.
4. Urges the patient to confront her husband with the problem promptly and then consoles her with the idea that, once she does, her marriage may be in great difficulty. It may well be, but any referral at this time is premature because there are no real data concerning Mrs. Bennett's personal plans for dealing with the situation. In reference to one-to-one relationships, it is well to remember that an errant partner can so move the other with acts of contrition that a second honeymoon instead of separation, may be sparked.

THE PATIENT WITH A VENEREAL DISEASE—Part II

After Mrs. Bennett had been given the opportunity to ventilate some of her feelings about having syphilis, Nurse Harrison administered the prescribed penicillin injection. The discussion then focused on the necessity of later blood studies, and a follow-up appointment was planned. The nurse explained to the patient that, because syphilis is a highly infectious communicable disease and a major threat to health if untreated, the law requires that all cases be reported to the department of health and that the purpose of reporting was to assist individuals who have been in contact with someone having the infection to receive medical attention. The nurse then asked Mrs. Bennett if she had given any thought to how she would discuss the matter with her husband. Her initial reaction was silence, broken only by the soft tapping of her right foot. Then, hesitantly, she said, "I have heard that you can get venereal disease in many different ways besides sexual relations. I am right, am I not?"

Which reply(ies) by Nurse Harrison would *most* likely constitute a *barrier* to therapeutic communication?

_____ 1. "No matter how the organism was transmitted, it does not change the fact that all contacts need to be treated."
_____ 2. "I am somewhat unclear about what you mean. Please elaborate more specifically."
_____ 3. "I seem to hear you saying that you have doubts about the way you became infected."
_____ 4. "You have heard of other ways of contacting syphylis? I am sure that is true, but almost everyone knows that the most common way is through sexual intercourse."

Discussion

1. Would inhibit communication because it is out of touch with what the patient seems to be experiencing emotionally and intellectually. Nonverbally Mrs. Bennett has indicated that she is still anxious and tense. Silences often are used to suppress feelings that are intolerable, and in this instance the patient seems to find it difficult to deal with the possibility of her husband's extramarital sexual activities. Had she been able or wanted to formulate a response to the nurse's question, Mrs. Bennett had ample opportunity to do so. When the patient broke her silence and changed the subject, her verbalization was of personal relevance and more representative of her needs at the moment—a need to move to a safer topic as a means of coping with a diminished self-esteem. The nurse has neglected to evaluate the meaning of the patient's total message and hence Mrs. Bennett's readiness to make use of information given. As a consequence, communication may be cut off because the data does not yet seem applicable to the patient's current assessment of her situation.

2. Would enhance the communication process because feedback asking for examples or illustrations tends to have the same effect as requesting the patient to tell more. Feedback or this type of perceptual check also conveys interest, a necessary condition for meaningful self-disclosures. Encouraging Mrs. Bennett to share what she has learned about the mode of transmission of syphilis provides the nurse with a natural opportunity for patient education, as well as a means of bringing the discussion back to the initial topic. Misconceptions about methods of contacting syphilis, such as sitting on a toilet seat or holding hands with an infected individual, may be cleared up. By acknowledging to the patient that it is possible to contact syphilis if you kiss an individual who has an oral infection, the nurse may reassure Mrs. Bennett that her contribution to the discussion is meaningful. The need for medical supervision of contacts could be presented in a different manner. Telling the patient that syphilis has been known to be spread in an innocuous fashion and that it often mimics many less serious diseases in the early stages may make the subject less threatening. Nurse Harrison, guided by the patient's responses, might then reiterate that the organism causing syphilis must be killed to prevent irreparable mental and physical harm.

3. May also keep the channels of communication open. The technique of paraphrasing is used to restate the cognitive content of the patient's message in a manner that captures the feeling tone of her body language. The patient's hesitancy in speaking and her nonverbal behavior may indicate a need to retain the image of her husband as a faithful marital partner and to deny the reality of her situation

for just a little longer. The topic that the patient has brought up is merely a circuitous route to responding to the nurse's original question. Following the patient's lead with acceptance and understanding is essential to helping her to gain a productive perspective of the problem and to move toward some resolution.

4. Is an example of how the technique of reflection may be misused to convey a critical comment. This response may be an expression of the nurse's annoyance at the change of subject, rather than an attempt to help the patient. Implicit in the fourth reply is belittlement of Mrs. Bennett's message and Mrs. Bennett herself as being uninformed. The patient is already in emotional pain, and approaches that are insensitive to her discomfort are most certain to terminate meaningful dialogue.

THE PATIENT WHO MAKES SEXUAL OVERTURES—Part I

Paul Hartman, a 23-year-old cabdriver, sustained severe spinal cord injury 2 months ago as a result of a diving accident in a friend's backyard pool. The extensive upper motor neuron lesion caused paralysis of his lower extremities, as well as disturbed bladder and bowel control. There is a serious doubt at this time whether he will be able to experience coitus or sire children. Intensive physiotherapy has helped to develop the upper part of his body, so that he is able to do many things with his arms. Paul recently had a spinal fusion operation preparatory to learning how to ambulate with braces and crutches and is currently confined to bed. Such nursing activities as assisting him with personal hygiene, skin care, dressing changes, positioning, and turning require the staff to spend a great deal of time at his bedside. Even though he has made remarkable physical progress, his psychologic condition remains stormy, although frank expressions of shock, disbelief, remorse, and anger are somewhat less frequent. Communications of a sexual nature now seem to engage most of his psychic energies. He spends a great deal of time poring over magazines with pictures of nude women, openly making comparisons between the pictures and female personnel and bragging in vulgar terms about his past sexual prowess.

Today, when Nurse Mahoney approaches to take his temperature, Paul leers at her and says, "Every time you come near me, my temperature rises; I bet you're one of those hot little Florence Nightingales I've heard about. There is nothing the doctors around here can do that I can't do better. Close the door, and I'll show you just what I mean."

Which reply to Paul by Nurse Mahoney would probably be the *most* appropriate?

_____ 1. "That was some monologue, Paul. You seem to be in a mood for conversation. I have a feeling that you still have many unanswered questions in your mind about your accident. Is this a fair statement? If you need more privacy for discussion, you can have it."

_____ 2. "Some part of that greeting was probably meant to be a compliment. However, the nature of your conversation indicates that like many males you have the usual stereotypes about nurses. Since the lack of privacy doesn't seem to be an inhibiting factor, the door can stay open while we explore some of these misconceptions further."

_____ 3. "You seem to be in good spirits today and are obviously feeling better. Tell me if I am wrong, but what I think you are really saying right now is that you have many self-doubts about your masculinity and sexual adequacy. If you feel you can talk about this better with the door closed, then I'll close it."

_____ 4. "Everything one hears and chooses to believe does not make a suitable topic for conversation. Under the circumstances it may be best to have Mr. Leary, the male nurse, either take your temperature from now on or at least be present when I do so."

Discussion

1. Is the most appropriate because it shows the best understanding of human sexuality and perhaps of Paul's needs at this time. When future hopes and dreams are instantaneously demolished, the processes of reconstructing a new self-image and of resocialization are long and arduous. Part of the self-image is one's sexuality. Human sexuality is not restricted to physical sex acts or propaganda about them. Human sexuality is expressed in every aspect of one's life-style: clothing, car, occupation, hobbies, and interpersonal relationships. Thus, nursing intervention does not have to be based on a direct response to the sexual content of Paul's message. Anxiety concerning his job, housing, recreation, relationship with family and friends, and other practical problems of everyday life may be so intense that these matters cannot be broached directly. The first response seems consistent with the best efforts of the nurse to ascertain and validate her assessment of Paul's immediate needs without *further* damage to his precarious self-concept. If his concerns relate solely to sexual functioning, the nurse can expand her helping capacities by suggesting sources of information or offering to make inquiries on his behalf from consultants in the field.

2. Is an approach not to be recommended because it allows for too much misinterpretation on the patient's part. Without insulting or embarrassing Paul, the nurse must communicate to him that the relationship

is a professional one for shared problem solving and not an opportunity for him to open his Pandora's box of sexual fantasies. This is especially important when the possibility exists that the nurse, personally, may become a central figure in his fantasy world and a target for his affectionate feelings. By encouraging Paul to clarify his "misconceptions," which he will no doubt do with the utmost dedication, the nurse sets the stage for an intimacy from which it may prove difficult to extricate herself. If she becomes the love object of the patient's pent-up emotions, she may well become the part of Paul's problem most painful to resolve.

3. Is also defensible and involves the technique of interpreting or reflecting the basic meaning of Paul's message without digging too deeply into his psyche. The nurse presents her ideas or understanding of the patient's communication in a *tentative* manner that permits Paul to respond to her statement and to continue the discussion if he chooses. The nurse needs to keep in mind that reflections of a sexual nature may intensify sexuality and that a sense of ease during the discussion will help keep the conversation productive. The success of this approach is also contingent on the existence of an interpersonal relationship that gives Paul sufficient ego support that he feels secure enough to disclose his feelings and attitudes about what has been said and what is happening to him. Next he may be slowly and gently assisted in exploring and examining his feelings. In this manner, both patient and nurse may gain a broader perspective of the problem and cooperatively seek solutions that foster growth and change.

4. Attends to the overt message while completely overlooking the possibility that a more meaningful covert message is being communicated. Possibly Paul is trying to defend against deep personal feelings of despair by making obvious and crude "passes" at the nurse. Nurses, as representatives of the female species, may also be representative test cases for Paul's attempts to reassure himself that he is still attractive or at least acceptable to the opposite sex. Paul fails the test when the nurse not only rejects the subject of sex as being taboo but also threatens to punish him for having such preoccupations. This approach may serve to emphasize the patient's disabilities and foreclose his hopes of reestablishing some equilibrium between himself and his environment. Basic to successful nursing intervention in this kind of patient-care situation is a sense of ease with one's own sexuality and an awareness of the fragility of the patient's self-image as the nurse attempts to guide the conversation to more fruitful areas of discussion. There is yet another possibility. Words can be used for their shock value with the manipulative purpose of not only keeping the conversation superficial but also of driving the

listener away. Perhaps the nurse reacted exactly as Paul intended. In conclusion, rejecting the patient and his pass may be an overreaction quite disproportionate to the amount of discord in the situation.

THE PATIENT WHO MAKES SEXUAL OVERTURES—Part II

Prior to the accident, Paul had his own apartment, and intensive rehabilitation is required before he will again be self-sufficient. He has progressed to the point where he is able to transfer himself into and out of a wheelchair and manage self-care with less nursing assistance. During his long period of confinement to bed, Paul has found that, by tugging on his Foley catheter and looking at erotic pictures, he is able to achieve a psychogenic erection. Physicians have explained to Paul that no definitive prognostic statements concerning his sexual functioning can be made at this time. Whether he is in or out of bed, masturbation has become such a dominant part of his behavioral pattern that Paul refuses to mingle with other patients and has become resourceful in finding reasons for staff members to come into his room. If the personnel are women, Paul openly manipulates himself in their presence. Because of this, there is a great deal of reluctance even to answer his call light. A team conference is held, attended by professional as well as paraprofessional staff involved in the patient's care. The objectives are to understand the ramifications of paraplegia from Paul's point of view, to resolve problems related to nursing care, and to discuss plans for rehabilitation. However, it soon becomes evident that the predominant area of concern is Paul's masturbatory habits. After a lively discussion, the group seems evenly divided between two proposals: (1) nursing intervention that is *accepting* of Paul's behavior and (2) nursing intervention that is *rejecting* of Paul's behavior. You are uncommitted and your opinion represents the deciding factor, or the vote that will break the deadlock. In accordance with the basic tenets of the team conference, approaches arrived at by group consensus will be uniformly adopted.

After you have weighed the varying points of view presented by each side, which position would you support as the *most* appropriate?

_____ 1. For nursing intervention that is *accepting* of Paul's behavior.
_____ 2. For nursing intervention that is *rejecting* of Paul's behavior.

Discussion

1. Those who favor nursing measures conveying *acceptance* of Paul's behavior argue that sex is one of the basic human needs. Preconceptions about how an individual should express this need when socially approved outlets are no longer available lead to biased courses of action that may be in the staff's rather than the patient's best interest. Sex is an integral part of the human experience and is more prolife

than abject resignation to one's physical limitations. Behavior that seems deviant may be the norm for a particular disabled person, and nurses may need to learn to live with a broader range of sexual behavior than is usually acceptable in a therapeutic relationship.

Because of what Paul has had to cope with, masturbation may be a badly needed emotional corroboration of his manliness. To limit his opportunity to experiment with a form of expression of his sexuality or to communicate to him that masturbation is unacceptable in a professional relationship may increase his sexual anxiety or fears of sexual inadequacy. This, in turn, may create problems in his rehabilitation, one goal of which is acquiring confidence in his ability to form a loving relationship with another human being. Other than explaining to Paul that trauma caused by tugging on his catheter may predispose him to a bladder infection, the staff need not call attention to his behavior but support his struggles with a lowered self-image by increasing the frequency of communications, whether he is masturbating or not. This seems to be the best way to help Paul to find equilibrium within himself, as well as his environment. Then, too, Paul's masturbation is probably a transient means of release of tension, a form of self-consolation as a defense against isolation and loneliness. The practice will most likely become self-limiting once other aspects of his rehabilitation claim his attention. Calling attention to or interfering with the patient's masturbatory pattern before alternative tension-releasing opportunities are found is to deprive him of the psychologic encouragement he may need to regain a sense of wholeness.

To sum up, because Paul's behavior is nonconformist, the staff have made him the target of their anxiety, and rejection of his behavior is a means of meeting their, rather than the patient's needs. If Paul is confronted with such feelings in persons on whom he must depend, inner resources required to face and discuss his need for help probably will be diverted toward defending himself against the helpers.

2. The proponents of "setting limits" on Paul's behavior counter that his cooperation with his rehabilitation program to date and his demonstrable progress indicate his interest in learning to live as normal a life as possible. Part of a normal life is some degree of conformity to the restrictions imposed by society on sexual behavior. Nursing personnel abdicate their responsibility when they fail to set limits on behavior that may prove maladaptive outside a health care setting. Although recognizing the depth and extent of Paul's frustrations with his life situation and his profoundly altered self-image, the staff also need to be diligent in discouraging behavior that may lead to further disequilibrium. The patient will not feel cared for if no one cares

enough to communicate to him the truth about his behavior and to offer assistance to help him control his uninhibited impulses.

Helpers can be empathetic and try to experience what Paul is feeling without themselves feeling powerless or compelled to respond in ways that might impede the patient's progress toward living a self-satisfying life. True, Paul has suffered a catastrophic disability, but he need not become further disabled by sexual behavior certain to add to adjustive difficulties in forming meaningful human relationships. If the staff do not have reasonable expectations for his conformity to social standards, they risk communicating to Paul that he is socially substandard and thus lacking in capacity for health growth and change.

The point is neither to leave the behavior unnoticed nor to dwell on it. Somewhere in between the two extremes, planned nursing activities may be devised to assist the patient in overcoming the behavior.

Perhaps after a mutual exploration of the goals of nursing intervention, some form of behavior modification may be carried out. Paul can be given a choice: the staff will freely communicate with him when he is not masturbating and limit conversation when he is. In contrast to exploiting the patient-care situation, Paul is encouraged in his abilities to react effectively in achieving equilibrium within himself and between himself and the staff. A consistent belief in his ability to respond in health-facilitating ways may communicate to the patient the worth that the staff sees in him and give him the support needed to develop it in socially adaptive ways.

In summary, adjustments to catastrophic illness create complex emotional problems, but the staff need not permit such problems to become chronic.

•   •   •

What did you decide? If you have a great deal of difficulty in making up your mind, perhaps Henderson's definition of nursing on p. 4 will be helpful.

DOCTOR-NURSE CONFLICT

Mrs. Kruger, a thin 62-year-old woman with cardiovascular disease, attends the medical clinic monthly for treatment of hypertension. Today she came to the clinic prior to her scheduled appointment complaining of headaches and dizziness of 4 days' duration. Miss Petrie, the medical screening nurse, found that Mrs. Kruger had not been adhering to her medication regimen and was using salt more liberally in her diet than she should. In a discussion of this with the patient, Mrs. Kruger claimed that she usually felt no different when she did than when she did not. Miss Petrie took the patient's blood pressure and began to explore with her the relationships among her medications, diet, and the control of high blood pressure. When Mrs. Kruger asked the nurse what her blood pressure reading was, Nurse Petrie informed her that it was 180/94. After the screening visit the patient was examined by Dr. Colbert, who assured her that everything was satisfactory and that no change was needed in her therapy. Mrs. Kruger became upset, telling the physician that anyone with her symptoms and a blood pressure of 180/94 certainly needed to have new medications prescribed. Considerable time was required for Dr. Colbert to mollify the patient and persuade her to leave the clinic. Mrs. Kruger, however, was receptive to referral by the doctor to the visiting nurse service for supervision of her health care regimen in her home setting. After the patient's departure Dr. Colbert approached Nurse Petrie and loudly berated her for giving the patient medical information that upset her and led to an intolerable scene. He further admonished the nurse not to intrude on the doctor-patient relationship in such a way again. Without giving Nurse Petrie time to respond, Dr. Colbert stalked away. Taken back and extremely embarrassed, Nurse Petrie went to the lounge to regain her composure.

When Nurse Petrie returns to the clinical area, how do you think she should *initiate* the problem-solving process?

_____ 1. Nurse Petrie should ignore Dr. Colbert's belligerent attitude and calmly continue to exercise her own professional approach to comprehensive care.

_____ 2. Nurse Petrie should request Dr. Colbert to accompany her when he is free to the administrative offices, where professional representatives of both disciplines can listen objectively and help clear up the role misconceptions.

_____ 3. Nurse Petrie should tell Dr. Colbert that she didn't appreciate his remonstrances and would like to discuss the matter in private at his earliest convenience.

_____ 4. Nurse Petrie should arrange a group conference for nursing personnel in the various clinics to ascertain if this is an isolated incident or a pattern of physician behavior necessitating a collegial response.

Discussion

1. Is a form of nonverbal communication that seems to be a kind of immobilization in the face of an important issue. To remain silent when one's integrity is attacked is to bottle up resentment that may adversely affect personal as well as professional functioning. What is worse, Dr. Colbert may interpret Nurse Petrie's silence as deference to the higher position that physicians enjoy in employing institutions.

There is also a greater risk in deliberately ignoring the presence of another (said at times to be the cruelest form of nonverbal behavior), which is that Dr. Colbert may think that he had just cause: sullen nurses need to be berated and certainly not respected. Silent withdrawal will be helpful neither to the nurse nor to patients. She will feel little satisfaction in her work, and patients may become ill at ease in her presence.

2. Will not help the nurse to stand on her own two feet when necessary. It is preferable for the nurse to learn to deal with conflict in the context in which it occurs and involving initially only the immediate parties. Once a problem is given an arena, the need to maintain self-esteem becomes paramount. Defenses tend to become more pronounced and positions to harden in the presentation of "my side" and "your side." One-to-one dialogue is a beginning basis for better mutual understanding of each discipline. Following such understanding may be increased acceptance of each person's unique contribution. Certainly there is a need for administrative guidelines and interdisciplinary efforts to provide coordinated, consistent, and cooperative patient care. The communication between Nurse Petrie and Dr. Colbert need not be pleasant to be fruitful. A great deal will have been accomplished if mutual respect, essential to collaborative functioning, results from the nurse's communication efforts.

3. Would seem to initiate the problem-solving process best because Nurse Petrie is requesting an opportunity to explore the situation fully *before* deciding on a course of action. Nurses who consider themselves to be working in a peer relationship with physicians will not hesitate to express openly their concerns regarding problematic areas in patient care. An honest expression of feelings about the episode may communicate to the doctor that the nurse respects his ability to handle sincere comments and wants to improve the helping process in a manner that is in the best interest of patients. There are several difficulties in this situation that need to be sorted out. Does the physician really believe that patients have no right to know their blood pressure readings, or does he believe that informing them is the doctor's prerogative—sometimes or always? Does he understand that the nurse's choice was not an act of capriciousness, or could his blowup be his reaction to the last of a series of unfortunate events in a bad day? What all this means is that conflict cannot be resolved unless the channels of communication are kept open. There is also the probability that Nurse Petrie will gain a sense of mastery from having independently used her own resources and strengths in dealing with stresses of her professional life situation.

4. May only widen the controversy. Nurse Petrie and Dr. Colbert should

hold a "summit conference" first before Nurse Petrie "brings in the troops." Normally one does not involve peers in one's own personal conflicts or difficulties until one's full measure of competence has been used and the issue at stake has clear implications for the profession as a whole. It is more desirable that the individual nurse take the initiative in defining precisely what and how much can be done by her own efforts in resolving communication problems. This is the immediate goal. Although team efforts certainly would be needed to prevent future clashes in roles, the group discussion would need to be planned thoughtfully and interdisciplinarily if there were to be any meaningful dialogue and proposals concerning role definition.

A DANCING CAREER CUT SHORT—Part I

Beverly Haines, a 21-year-old ballet dancer, has been treated since the age of 19 for systemic lupus erythematosus, an inflammatory connective tissue disorder of unknown origin. She has had several periods of hospitalization in her hometown, and medical treatment seemed to keep the disease controlled or in a state of remission up to the present time. Because she was exhibiting signs of chronic renal failure, she was transferred to a renowned medical center for more intensive therapy; but dialysis at the center is proving futile in the face of the rapid progression of other symptoms. Beverly's therapeutic regimen consists mainly of comfort measures, and, in spite of her lethargy, headaches, itching skin, drowsiness, and marked loss of weight, she often expresses the belief that a successful means of medical intervention will be found. Prior to her illness Beverly shared a cooperative living arrangement with other members of her troupe. However, she was forced by financial as well as physical incapacities to return to live with her mother. Beverly's parents were divorced when she was 9 years of age; she was left in her mother's custody. The patient speaks lovingly of her mother and bitterly of her father. She seems to resent the fact that he remarried immediately after the divorce and started a new family. She states that the only contact she has with her father is an occasional "run in" at a dance concert, and her greeting to him is just barely cordial. However, most of her conversation with health personnel is about the period of her life when she was healthy and actively involved in her career. During one of these conversations with Nurse Martinez, Beverly remarked, "I have made up in my mind that because of my dancing background I am the type of person with the stamina to recover rapidly once the right combination of drugs is found."

Which approach by Nurse Martinez would probably be the most appropriate way of handling the patient's denial?

_____ 1. Establish eye contact with Beverly, take her hand, and say nothing.

_____ 2. Establish eye contact with the patient, pause, and then add, "Medical treatment cannot make you well, Beverly, but there may be many other things we can do to make you comfortable."

_____ 3. Sit down by her bedside, pat her gently on the shoulder, and explain that right now physicians have no way of helping her to overcome her sickness but that they are still trying hard through research to find one.

_____ 4. Sit down by her bedside, take her hand, and comment that, although the odds right now seem to be against her recovery, it is better for her to feel as she does than just to give up.

Discussion

1. Would probably be the most appropriate way of handling Beverly's denial, based on the following premises:
   a. Denial is a defense that dying patients use to escape the agonizing reality of their death.
   b. Denial is an avoidance technique designed to convey tacitly the need for threatening thoughts to remain unspoken.
   c. Denial must be reduced cautiously, lest the anxiety generated overtax tenuous coping capacities.
   d. Reduction of denial may be desirable because it allows the patient to release a multitude of troublesome feelings and share them. Sharing burdens may make them easier to bear.

   The first approach neither challenges nor reinforces the patient's denial but is a combination of therapeutic techniques that may convey compassion and encouragement for the patient to communicate on a deeper level if she wishes. Whereas a slightly raised eyebrow or a frown transmits a message of puzzlement or disagreement, a steady sympathetic gaze may communicate understanding of Beverly's unreadiness to personalize her death openly. However, silence and touch in conjunction with eye contact often convey, "I am here if you need me; I care." Silence will give both the patient and nurse an interlude in which to collect their thoughts. However, it should not persist to the extent that it adds to the patient's discomfort. The nurse may need to initiate further conversation by reflecting, "You have made up your mind . . ." or by injecting an open-ended phrase, for example, "You were saying. . . ." If Beverly is the first to break the silence, what she says will most likely be extremely significant. Moreover, because she does not have to react to the nurse's conclusions, Beverly may have sufficient emotional reserves to risk participation in the reduction of her denial. Most worthwhile in this situation may be a minimum of words and a maximum of warmth.

2. May cause too rapid a diminution of hope in a patient whose adaptive defenses against death seem to be a pattern of denial. Life is lived

in hope. Many hopes of individuals, either sick or well, are grossly unrealistic. Although it is wrong to reinforce false hope, removing all hope at once is not helpful, for without *some* hope that conditions will improve, life itself will have no meaning.

3. Is simply restatement of a truth that the patient has not expressed any need to know. Patients indicate by their communications the kinds of information that they want. Because Beverly is at an age when she has achieved some knowledge and mastery of life, she also has a knowledge of death and appreciates all that she is now losing in its rapid approach. The facade of denial covers feelings that may be totally intolerable; before she is willing, she should not be obliged to face the personal defeat of death. Beverly did not ask if she were dying; the reality of her situation certainly has not escaped her. Although the third response is a sensitive approach to the patient's denial, the informational content of the message may reinforce denial or break down emotional defenses. Neither outcome seems desirable under the circumstances.

4. Communicates contradictory messages. Beverly is being told that, although what she is thinking is wrong, it is right to be thinking that way. Since it is unlikely that she will seek clarification, either the entire message will have little meaning to her, or the confused meaning could arouse such deeply disturbing feelings that any productive communication would be precluded.

A DANCING CAREER CUT SHORT—Part II

Beverly's condition is deteriorating rapidly. Her mother visited a couple of days ago and plans to return as soon as possible, since the physicians notified her that the patient's respiratory pattern seemed characteristic of impending coma. Mrs. Haines contacted her former husband regarding the gravity of their daughter's illness. He was able to catch an earlier flight to the city and called the hospital from the airport to request that Beverly be informed of his imminent arrival. When Nurse Martinez relayed the message, the patient laboredly specified, "Do not let him in this room. I don't want to see him. Tell him to go back to his other children!"

Of the following courses of action, which one would probably be the *least* appropriate for Nurse Martinez to take?

_____ 1. Telling Beverly that she should reconsider the decision and that, if she then felt the same way, it would probably be better if she shared these feelings directly with her father.

_____ 2. Reassuring Beverly that, when her father arrives, if she still feels that this is definitely what she wants, the decision will be conveyed to him.

_____ 3. Telling Beverly that her father's desire to visit is a natural act of parental concern and that he needs to be given at least the opportunity to personally effect a reconciliation with his daughter.

_____ 4. Explaining to Beverly that this is one request that the nurse feels she does not wish to honor and exploring with Beverly the possibility of designating someone else—perhaps the head nurse, her physician, or the chaplain.

Discussion

1. Would be difficult *not* to choose, since anger is indigenous to the process of dying and a great deal may be directed against those whom the patient cares about and will miss. It is also true that approaching death often mitigates conflict and draws family members emotionally closer. Because one of the roles of the nurse is that of facilitator, she may also believe that facilitating the strengthening of familial bonds, especially when they are most slender, may enlarge the patient's support system of comfort and care. However, the nurse needs to be mindful that encouraging father and daughter confrontation may not be in the patient's best interest and that emerging feelings may cause further insult, rather than relief, to the patient's adaptive psychic resources.

2. Is supportable because Beverly, legally an adult, has the right to confer or withhold bedside privileges. A significant variable is that her attitude toward her father seems to be consistent and not a recent consequence of personality changes from the disease process. The nurse also has the role of professional intermediary between the patient and family. This puts a heavy responsibility on the nurse because in the role of intermediary it is almost impossible to suspend judgment about some of the patient's unique decisions. However, because the patient is the focus of the nursing process, helping her to meet her needs is the nurse's primary responsibility, and rarely will this be truer than in caring for a patient who has no future.

3. Would seem to be the least appropriate because the nurse, perhaps identifying with the father or with an idealistic concept of paternal feelings, is assigning positive motives to his actions without validation. Furthermore, she is using her value judgment to make an emotional appeal to the patient. Such appeals may be intimidating enough to arouse guilt, depression, or more anger. Although feelings of family members are extremely important, it is unfair to expect or urge the patient to consider the emotional comfort of others. Although some patients certainly elect to do so, others do not.

4. Is a different kind of example of genuineness. It does not give the nurse license to reveal whatever she pleases in patient-care situations

but rather is the disclosure of honest feelings for *constructive* reasons. Genuineness employed constructively is essential to maintaining trust. Sharing honest feelings with the patient may convey to her that she is a partner in the relationship; partners share in the decision-making process, although they do not have to agree with or carry out the decisions. The patient may not like the nurse's position but respect her directness. Knowing that the nurse can be depended on to be genuine in all her interactions with the patient and that she works with other members of the health team on the patient's behalf may make more secure Beverly's need to believe that she will always be comforted and cared for.

A FATHER MEETS HIS INFANT SON

Jason Sanford, 8 pounds, 6 ounces, and 21 inches in length, made his entrance into the world after 9 months' gestation via an uncomplicated vaginal delivery. His father, a postal clerk, was unable to be present during labor and delivery. Mrs. Sanford seemed proud of her son and exclaimed delightedly over him in the delivery room. When Mr. Sanford arrived at the hospital, his wife was sleeping soundly on the postpartal ward, and Jason was in the adjacent nursery. After finding out from Nurse Morrison that his wife was doing well, Mr. Sanford decided not to disturb her and excitedly requested to see his son. The nurse escorted the father to the nursery and stayed with him as he stared at the newborn intently through the window. Shaking his head from side to side, Mr. Sanford turned to Nurse Morrison to declare, "That is about the ugliest baby I've ever seen in my life!"

After she recovers her composure, which reply by Nurse Morrison probably shows the *most* astute assessment of the situation?

_____ 1. "We all tend to use differently even words we are all familiar with. Please tell me exactly what you mean by *ugly*."
_____ 2. "Some babies have a little more difficulty being born than others, and this often accounts for an unusual appearance at birth."
_____ 3. "I can see that you are concerned. Let's unwrap little Jason for a closer inspection; then more than likely you will change your mind."
_____ 4. "Obviously something is upsetting you. Let me explain what most newborns look like, and then you will see that Jason is perfectly normal."

Discussion

1. Would seem to be the most astute assessment of the situation: the nurse is aware that she needs clarification of Mr. Sanford's choice of words to understand the situation better from his point of view.

For example, if fathers remark, "That is about the meanest (or baddest) baby I've ever seen," in some parts of the country, they mean the *greatest:* far from being derogatory, they are the ultimate expressions of approval. Although it may be somewhat farfetched, it is possible that the term *ugly* may have cultural connotations unknown to the nurse. Even so, no clear communication seems possible until Mr. Sanford is encouraged either to define or further elaborate the meaning of his declaration. This is definitely not a time for guessing.

2. Nurse Morrison furnishes her own ideas about the father's reaction after *assuming* she knows what he means, or what is the actual source of his concerns. If the father is anxious, he may find it less than reassuring that the nurse thinks that his son is "unusual" or somehow different. In the second response Nurse Morrison, in a sense, is commiserating with Mr. Sanford, and if she communicates in any way to the father that she finds his son varies from the norm, her attitude may impede, rather than enhance, the father-son relationship.

3. May suggest to Mr. Sanford that his first opinion of his son is not a valid one and that some revision is in order. Therefore he is going to be given the immediate opportunity to change his mind. The problem with this approach is that Nurse Morrison seems unable to accept the father's authentic and individualistic expression. Hence Mr. Sanford is not helped to divulge specifically what is on his mind.

4. Nurse Morrison attends to the father's nonverbal communication and then directs the conversation to more neutral and familiar ground. Probably as a means of alleviating her anxiety she focuses on an area over which she has control. The father did not imply that Jason was abnormal: he said that his son was ugly. Parents usually don't express such feelings directly, but this one did, and this is what the nurse must deal with rather than offer a dissertation.

THE CRYING PATIENT

Mr. Couzman is a 42-year-old tax accountant who had a temporary ileostomy done several months ago because of severe attacks of ulcerative colitis that proved unresponsive to medical intervention. He is being readmitted to the surgical ward because the diseased part of his bowel has healed sufficiently to allow for reconstructive surgery, and he will no longer have to contend with the liquid fecal evacuations through an opening in his abdomen. Mr. Couzman is an affable, attractive patient who gained the admiration of the staff because of his motivation and success in learning self-care rather quickly. After an exchange of warm greetings all around, Nurse Wilson settled the patient in his room; when she left, he was sitting up in bed reading the newspaper. Sometime later, Mrs. Wilson returned to discuss with him the preoperative nursing procedures. Although the curtains were drawn around his bed, through a partial opening the nurse observed him huddled in bed, his body turned toward the wall. Even though he had pulled the covers partially over his head, his soft weeping was audible. Sensing that someone was present, the patient momentarily turned his head toward the nurse but said nothing.

Which communication by Nurse Wilson probably shows the *best* understanding of the patient's needs at this time?

_____ 1. "I noticed that you were crying, Mr. Couzman. Here are some tissues. I will stay with you while you freshen up. Once your bed is made and the curtains drawn back, you'll probably feel a little better."

_____ 2. "Perhaps you would like to be left alone for the time being. I am going to leave now, but I'll be back in a short while."

_____ 3. "It is very human to cry when you are troubled. What's the matter? Did someone do or say something to upset you?"

_____ 4. "You have been through a lot, Mr. Couzman. Things won't get worse now. When you feel sad, try to think ahead to the life you'll be able to lead after surgery."

Discussion

1. Indicates that the nurse thinks that she must take direct action when confronted with turbulent emotions. Offering tissues to the patient may communicate that he should stop crying or put an end to his display of emotion. She implicitly reinforces her message by directing her attention to the physical aspects of the situation, rather than the emotional needs of the person involved. Intervention that prematurely stems the flow of tears may inhibit the patient from making use of an important, available avenue for expression of strong feelings. In the first communication the nurse does not use her presence as an effective means of support. Quietly staying with Mr. Couzman for a while might have been a preferable mode of communication. However, the length of time spent with him must take into account that human beings need privacy, as well as personal contact. Meaningful nursing approaches are flexible. In this society, right or wrong, males feel that they are weak or unmanly if they express themselves through tears. Therefore they may risk being real only in solitude. Crying has many meanings; it is not always a plea for help from others. There is the possibility that Mr. Couzman feels inwardly secure enough now to release the pent-up anxieties and frustrations involved in living with an ileostomy and maintaining the public image of self-reliance and control that he presents. The nurse may better sustain his efforts to gain equilibrium by giving more thought to the

possibility that Mr. Couzman may need to experience a state of separateness, as we all do at times, and retain his sense of masculinity by "unburdening" himself in private. The patient who feels that sincere attempts have been made to understand him may also feel comforted and cared for in his solitude.

2. Would seem to show the best understanding of the situation, although based on the assumption that the nurse is not seeking to avoid an emotional encounter of significance to the client. Assessment of the patient's nonverbal behavior and sensitivity to its dynamics seems to indicate that Mr. Couzman is trying to be alone. The drawn curtains, position in bed, and avoidance of eye-to-eye contact may be a means of setting up social distance and limiting interpersonal interaction. Notwithstanding the importance of such techniques of therapeutic communication as availability and listening, patients often require time away from others to get in touch with their real selves. The result of such efforts may be increased capacity to use the help that is offered. In this situation, it may be more therapeutic to keep the interaction brief and not call attention to behavior observed in an unguarded moment. Further regard for the patient's self-esteem may be shown by shielding him from intrusion and needless exposure of his vulnerability to others. This may be done by Nurse Wilson's communicating to the staff the pertinent aspects of her experience and indicating that Mr. Couzman seems to want to be by himself for a while. Smith* points out that exposure, whether physical, emotional, or both, can cause a patient considerable humiliation and distress. When the patient has lost his usual control and ability to "cover his nakedness," the nurse should assist him in "reclothing himself" with compassion, respect, and regard for his privacy.

3. Seeks an explanation of overt behavior that the patient may be unable or unwilling to supply in a rational, straightforward manner. If he has no conscious reasonable explanation to offer, he may conclude that his behavior is inappropriate; and, if he has a reason, he may hesitate to verbalize it, feeling that his explanation for violation of a larger, accepted social norm may be inadequate. Of key importance, however, is the principle that patients demonstrating a need for physiologic and psychologic *privacy* should not be encouraged to make self-disclosures that they may later regret. The patient whose self-structure seems built on self-control may experience feelings of self-deprecation after the divulgence of highly personal data that he really preferred to remain unknown. When the patient regains his

*Smith, D.: Patienthood and its threat to privacy, American Journal of Nursing **69**:508-513, 1969.

poise, he may come to resent the nurse who heard his disclosures when his defenses were down and be uncomfortable in her presence.

4. Nurse Wilson may be attempting to minimize her feelings of discomfiture. In attempting to defend against the anxieties and sense of inadequacy aroused by the crying patient, she suggests that the way to overcome strong emotions is to rise above or suppress them. By encouraging Mr. Couzman to present a front, or maintain a facade, the nurse also increases the probability that the patient will stop behavior that threatens her equilibrium. Furthermore, suppressed emotions do not disappear; they may reemerge in a disguised form that could be detrimental to the patient. We want the patient neither to suppress honest emotions nor to engage in behavior that may estrange him from his real self. The *crux* of this situation is discerning the conditions under which he may therapeutically get in touch with his deepest emotions.

THE PATIENT WHO FEARS LIFE MORE THAN DEATH

Mr. Kellerman, 30 years of age, is an insurance salesman who developed a progressive and irreversible loss of kidney function. The clinical course of his disease could first be controlled by adherence to strict diet, limitation of fluids, and adjustments of medication. When the symptoms of kidney failure could no longer be managed with conservative treatment, Mr. Kellerman was started on dialysis and, with his fiancée's assistance, learned the mechanics well enough to carry out the procedure at home. During the 18 months that he was on dialysis, several episodes of surgical intervention were needed to find suitable sites for shunts and fistulas for inserting the tubing that connected the patient to the machine. Because of the patient's insomnia, chronic daytime fatigue, and the time-consuming necessity of dialysis three times weekly, he worked on a part-time basis, and his earnings decreased considerably. He was accepted as a transplant candidate; during the interim between his acceptance and the availability of a cadaver kidney, he and his fiancée made tentative plans to marry. He has informed her and the treatment team, headed by Dr. Spellman, that if surgery is unsuccessful he will be unable to endure either further passive submission to the machine or the stringent medical regimen. The health team has had many interviews with Mr. Kellerman to help him consider carefully his solution to unsuccessful surgery and to weigh this solution against other possible alternatives. His fiancée has assured him that she is willing to face the future with him, come what may, but he feels that, if he is unable to live a normal life, it would be unfair to tie her to an "invalid." Mr. Kellerman underwent a transplantation procedure as planned, but, in spite of vigorous immunosuppressive therapy, signs of tissue rejection of the grafted kidney became evident. When Dr. Spellman discussed with the patient the necessity for immediate resumption of dialysis, Mr.

Kellerman explained that he meant it when he said that he could never again reconcile himself to having his lifeline intertwined with a machine and therefore, after having given the matter considerable thought, he was refusing all further treatment. After a long conversation and sharing of various points of view, the physician left to consult with the chaplain whom Mr. Kellerman had requested to see. Nurse Quinn, who was present during the discussion, remained with the patient.

She sat down by the patient's bedside, and after a brief silence Mr. Kellerman said, "From some of the things I heard you mention a while ago, I gather that you have had a lot of experience taking care of patients with complete kidney shutdown. I'll bet there is not too much that can be done for the poor devils in the end, is there?"

Which one of the following responses by Nurse Quinn would probably *preclude* meaningful dialogue about the patient's decision?

_____ 1. "I know that patients who have had profound disappointments, as you have, carry heavy burdens. There will be people around, as I am now, who will offer to share them."

_____ 2. "Yes, I have taken care of a lot of very sick people, and each human being is different. Try to let me know more about what you are thinking and feeling, so that I can answer your questions more specifically."

_____ 3. "I can appreciate your concern, but we never take for granted that there is nothing more to do. Although it is less difficult to help the patient who choses to cope, no patient is ever neglected."

_____ 4. "Let me see if I understand you correctly. It sounds to me as if you are wondering if dying will be painful and whether you'd be left all alone. Am I on the right track?"

Discussion

1. Implements the concept of caring. It responds to the apprehensive feeling tone of the patient's message that in the "nothing-more-to-do" stage of terminal illness he may be abandoned, or deserted. Caring is the essence of patient care throughout the life continuum, but it may be the crux of this kind of patient-care situation. Jourard has stated that "a person lives in response to the experience of repeated invitations to continue living."* Caring may "invite" Mr. Kellerman to pull himself into the future because it communicates that *he* has meaning and value, even though he believes that his life has none.

---

*From Jourard, S. M.: Living and dying. Suicide: an invitation to die, American Journal of Nursing **70**:269-275, 1970.

Caring provides human sustenance and may encourage the patient to explore further possibilities of discovering new purposes for living. Caring seems a prerequisite if the will to live is to take precedence over the will to die. In addition, caring also recognizes the patient's right to die with dignity if death be his rational choice.

2. Implements the concept of respect. Respect involves the commitment to try to understand the patient's situation so that the nurse can more effectively respond to his personal needs. Respect includes acknowledging that each human being must be seen as a unified whole who experiences his existence uniquely. Respect may be the catalyst to facilitate patient self-disclosure, so that the nurse can anticipate and work with him to alleviate some of the stresses inherent in the dying experience. The interest and concern communicated in this approach may reassure the patient that he is a worthy human being whose needs in the final stages of life will not be neglected.

3. Is not a sensitive response to a patient who has just refused permission for dialysis. The inference is that the patient's decision is based more on cowardice than on rational self-determination. The patient who seeks to control his destiny by refusing dialysis may arouse deeply disturbing conflict in the staff. Patients like Mr. Kellerman present the staff with an "emotional stimulus that triggers the most profound fear experienced in human life; that is, fear of death."* The patient wants to express his feelings and to have them accepted, but Nurse Quinn is unable or unwilling to participate in an experience wherein the acceptance of feelings threatens her self-preservative instinct. When dormant notions of immortality are belied, there seems to be some inherent disposition to produce change in the patient in the direction in which the helper feels *she* can most comfortably cope.

4. Is a candid perceptual check on the meaning of the patient's message and lets him know that one of the persons most likely to be involved in his care is not afraid to take a good look at what seems to be immediately troubling him. The nurse does not superimpose her ideas of appropriateness and inappropriateness concerning the patient's decision on the conversation but focuses, as he does, on the interim between his decision and death. Mr. Kellerman seems not to fear death but rather dying. (Will it be painful? How long will it take?) However, most of all he seems to be wondering if his final human experience will be devoid of dignity and human contact. He may want to have a normal diet and his friends around him—to define his life in terms of his own humanness. It is not difficult to understand some

*From Anger, D., and Anger, D. W.: Dialysis ambivalence: a matter of life and death, American Journal of Nursing **76:**276-277, 1976.

of the pressures that caused him to evaluate his life as meaningless; now we must value him as we try to understand the way that he chose to cope.

THE ALCOHOLIC

Mr. Patterson is a 42-year-old, socially prominent business executive who has had three previous hospitalizations within the last 7 months. Two admissions related to severe gastrointestinal complaints, and the third was for treatment of superficial injuries received in a minor car accident. His current hospitalization is for treatment of a fractured left wrist sustained in a fall down a flight of stairs at home. The physician has indicated on the patient's chart that the accident was preceded by a blackout, and a laboratory test showed raised blood alcohol levels. Mr. Patterson's left forearm is placed in a cast, and he will be discharged in 48 hours. His therapeutic regimen does not require the professional nurse to spend more than 10 to 15 minutes with him at least four times daily. Mr. Patterson is witty, cooperative, and warmly appreciative of any nursing attention that he receives. Laughter usually emanates from his room whenever visitors or staff are present. He jokes about the help that he needs with his bath and attributes the tremulousness of his hand when brushing his teeth to "bottle fatigue." He is apologetic because the procedure takes so long and becomes visibly agitated when he spills water on himself.

In reference to Mr. Patterson's alcoholism, which approach by the nurse is most likely to facilitate therapeutic communication?

_____ 1. "Mr. Patterson, there is something that I wish to talk over with you. I would like to get your feelings about the possibility that your drinking pattern is pronounced enough to cause some of the physical problems you are experiencing."

_____ 2. "Mr. Patterson, you are beginning to recover nicely from your fall. I don't wish to embarrass you, but your problem is not humorous. Here is some literature regarding Alcoholics Anonymous and other community resources available to help people with problems such as yours."

_____ 3. "I notice that you make a lot of jokes about drinking, Mr. Patterson; yet you seem embarrassed over your inability to control your hand movements. It seems apparent that alcoholism is causing you difficulties that you are reluctant to discuss."

_____ 4. "Mr. Patterson, there is something that I think you should know. Alcoholism ranks as the fourth major public health problem in the United States. It involves such elements as loss of control and interference with normal functioning, which are present in your pattern of hospitalization. The misuse of alcohol is a serious problem that we need to discuss."

Discussion

1. Would seem to be the most appropriate. This approach encourages
active partnership in the problem-solving process. When the patient
is encouraged to perceive relationships for himself, he may make
a more realistic assessment of the facts and recognize to some degree
that he has a drinking problem. Until Mr. Patterson admits that his
drinking is a problem, he is unlikely to consider reality-oriented
solutions. The nurse cannot help the alcoholic patient unless he sees
a need for the help she can provide. Genuine, appropriately timed
expressions of concern on the part of the nurse may communicate
to the patient that he is worthwhile human being with a disability
that can be overcome.

2. Seems inappropriate for two reasons. First, the nurse seems to disregard the fact that individuals can worry out loud in many ways.
"Cracking" jokes and the use of biting humor may be defenses against
anxiety, as well as the language of denial. It would be more therapeutic
to accept Mr. Patterson as he presents himself at this time: a vulnerable patient trying to cope with his fears through laughter and conviviality. Second, the nurse may be projecting personal feelings of discomfort concerning the subject of alcoholism on the patient. Telling
Mr. Patterson that she does not wish to embarrass him may communicate that alcoholism is something unmentionable, rather than
a legitimate psychosocial illness. In addition, pamphlets and related
literature are much more meaningful in reinforcing points previously
discussed or as a basis for future discussion.

3. Seems inappropriate because, although confrontation is a useful
therapeutic technique, Mueller* suggests that with the alcoholic
patient this approach is most likely to be constructive subsequent
to the establishment of a reasonably strong therapeutic relationship.
A primary objective is to help the patient to feel secure enough in
a relationship to discuss his problem with some degree of openness
and candor. To confront the patient prematurely with inconsistencies
between his verbal and nonverbal behavior may erode carefully
constructed defenses needed to protect a self-esteem already under
assault. Confrontation presents the individual with conclusions and
unless used with care may be perceived by the patient as a form
of entrapment badgering him into making a response. With an extremely vulnerable person this technique can contribute to self-depreciation and heighten feelings of futility. Under such circumstances,
therapeutic communication will be cut off. The client's concentration

*Mueller, J.: Treatment for the alcoholic: cursing or nursing, American Journal of Nursing
74:245-247, 1974.

on defending his ego may cause him to reject whatever help is proffered. This is a real possibility, since Mr. Patterson has already indicated that currently he needs to use humor as an outlet for his true concerns.

4. Presumes that the patient will first consent to be taught something he may already know and to respond in ways bound by the nurse's concept of appropriateness. This "pull-yourself-together-or-dire-things-will-happen" approach rarely moves individuals to marshall their resources in seeking solutions. If the patient does not share in the assessment of his problem, it is unrealistic to expect that he will accept responsibility for dealing with it. Strong appeals to fear are likely to be counterproductive. People strive for self-consistency, and ideas that aggravate their state of disequilibrium are apt to be disregarded.

GIFTS AND THE NURSE—Part I

Mrs. Mazor, a 28-year-old housewife, has been hospitalized for several weeks for treatment of overall joint pain due to rheumatoid arthritis. Because of the limited range of motion in all her joints, she cannot dress herself, comb her hair, or take more than a few steps without assistance. She spends a great deal of her time sitting in a wheelchair and looking out the window. She is married and the mother of two children, age 6 and 11. With rest, medication, and physiotherapy she is optimistic that she will soon be able to return home and take care of herself and her family again. On admission, she refused to send home or place in the hospital safe the exquisite wide copper bracelet that she wears on her right arm. She states that she doesn't believe the bracelet has any special curative powers but that it is her "good luck piece." She is congenial and cooperative with all the staff but seems to have developed a special fondness for Nurse Pernell, who handles and positions her with the utmost gentleness and compassion. This nurse admitted the patient to the unit and is often assigned to give her care. Mrs. Mazor also has high regard for Dr. Griffel, an intern involved with her medical regimen. One day she gives Nurse Pernell an expensive birthstone ring. Hospital policy specifies that the staff should not receive any form of remuneration from patients.

Under these circumstances, which response by Nurse Pernell seems *most* appropriate?

_____ 1. "Mrs. Mazor, I don't wish to seem ungrateful, but I must refuse the gift. Hospital policy strictly forbids nurses to accept any presents from patients."

_____ 2. "I am sorry, Mrs. Mazor. I would accept the lovely ring if I could. Even though I don't like some of the rules around here, I must follow them."

_____ 3. "The ring is gorgeous, Mrs. Mazor; but tell me, why do you feel it necessary to give me such an expensive gift?"

_____ 4. "What a beautiful gift, Mrs. Mazor! I'll have to check with administration to see whether I can keep it, but, even if it is mine for only a short time, I appreciate the thought."

Discussion

1. May be considered appropriate *if* the nurse heeds Hector's stern warning that "gifts in money or kind should not enter the nurse-patient relationship."[*] Hector believes that patients who tender gifts do so with the expectation of favors or preferential treatment. Gifts may be a manipulative means of gaining unfair advantage over other patients and establishing relationships with professional personnel for purely selfish ends. Even if the nurse were certain that the gift was prompted only by gratitude, it is still in the nature of a tip and demeaning to the concept of professionalism. However, nurses may also want to give some thought to the fact that gift giving is a significant form of nonverbal communication and that acceptance or rejection of gifts may hinge not so much on hospital policy per se as on communicating their assessment of the total patient-care situation to their immediate supervisors, few of whom are impervious to rational appeal if a rule may adversely affect therapeutic relationships. Instead of rejecting the gift outright, the nurse could indicate to Mrs. Mazor that she would find out if exceptions to the rule can be made. This approach, in addition to personal comments about the gift, would seem more gracious than to reiterate a policy in a manner that implies rebuke.
2. Differs significantly from the first; that is, the nurse acknowledges and refuses the gift in a manner that is much more sensitive to the patient's feelings. The nurse's brief disclosure of her feelings to the patient leaves little room for Mrs. Mazor to interpret the refusal of the gift as an act of personal rejection. Although I would not select this as the best response, it is certainly better than the first one.
3. May bring a highly intellectualized approach to a patient-care situation in which none is needed. Of course, all behavior is purposeful, and one could speculate endlessly on Mrs. Mazor's unconscious motivations. The gift could be a reaction formation to the hostility that the patient may feel toward a healthy nurse. Complications in her Oedipal complex may have given rise to homosexual tendencies and a need to seal a desired relationship symbolically with the customary ring. However, it is also true that every "tic and twitch" is not

---

[*]From Hector, W.: Modern nursing: theory and practice, London, 1960, William Heinemann, Ltd., p. 8.

psychologically suspect. Many behaviors are culturally conditioned. Gift giving on such occasions as holidays, birthdays, and anniversaries is a national custom, and gifts are much more meaningful at other times. The stability of social customs in new situations is essential to feelings of security. To have one's customs scrutinized and questioned with no demonstrable need may make it more difficult for the patient to fulfill the basic human need to belong—to be accepted.

4. Seems to be the most appropriate response. The nurse who gives of herself in a caring human relationship gives her most precious possession. Fromm has stated that such a person "cannot help but bring something to life in the other person—giving implies to make the other person a giver also, and they both share in the joy of what they have brought to life. . . ."* Far from being suspect, Mrs. Mazor's gift to Nurse Pernell may be a natural and human response to a supportive relationship. The personal satisfaction that comes from giving can at times be as therapeutic as the care the patient receives.

GIFTS AND THE NURSE—Part II

Aggressive treatment of Mrs. Mazor's arthritis has brought a partial remission of symptoms. Her muscle strength and range of motion have increased enough for her to use a walker in getting about her room. She employs a wheelchair on the infrequent occasions when she visits with other patients in the solarium at the end of the corridor. Mrs. Mazor has not been eating or sleeping well for the past 3 or 4 days, and it is difficult to get her to verbalize her feelings. Although salicylate and prednisone tablets seem to have given her a great deal of relief with relatively few side effects, Mrs. Mazor seems disappointed with the treatment outcome.

Instead of viewing her life as being complicated by a chronic condition, she has lately begun to speak of herself as a "hopeless cripple." She seemed little impressed when emphasis was placed on the skills that she does have and her positive accomplishments, but this afternoon she appears to be in a cheerful mood and manages to wave warmly to the staff as she passes the nurse's station going to and from the solarium.

One of the nursing assistants comments to the head nurse, Miss Debnaum, that Mrs. Mazor is not wearing her bracelet today. When Miss Debnaum enters Mrs. Mazor's room, the patient is gazing intently at her hands and unsuccessfully trying to bring her fingers together to make a fist.

In response to Nurse Debnaum's inquiry about the bracelet Mrs. Mazor lightly remarks that she removed the bracelet because it was becoming uncomfortable and interfered with her wrist movements. Furthermore, since

*From Fromm, Erich: The art of loving, New York, 1970, Bantam Books, Inc., pp. 20-21.

Dr. Griffel has admired the bracelet several times, she plans to give it to him when he makes his evening rounds.

Which of the following patient-nurse interactions would be the *most* insightful at this time?

_____ 1. "Mrs. Mazor, I know how fond you are of that bracelet. I have a feeling that giving up your good luck piece means that you now have more confidence in your medical regimen. You couldn't have picked a nicer person to give it to than Dr. Griffel. He is doing all that a doctor could do to make you well."

_____ 2. "I am concerned about your present condition. I have always had the feeling that under no circumstances would you part with your bracelet. I also notice that today you have been literally 'pacing the halls' in your wheelchair. I do not know exactly what all this means, but I am wondering whether you have been thinking of suicide."

_____ 3. "Mrs. Mazor, if the bracelet made you uncomfortable, you were wise to take it off. I know things haven't been going the way you hoped, but you have made remarkable improvement, and with continued therapy your arthritis will be less restrictive than you now seem to think."

_____ 4. "I have noticed that lately you haven't been eating or sleeping well, and today you just don't seem to be yourself. I am concerned that, feeling the way you do, you would part with a cherished possession. Something seems to be troubling you, but I don't know what. I am going to sit with you, and perhaps you may want to tell me what you mean when you say you are a hopeless cripple."

Discussion

1. Is a conclusion by the nurse that seems inconsistent with human nature and hence the least insightful approach. People are unlikely to tempt fate by giving up a good luck charm just when it is beginning to "work," or when they start showing signs of improvement. Rather, Mrs. Mazor's bracelet would assume even greater significance if she thought that therapy would bring her additional gains. Moreover, assessment of the patient's nonverbal behavior as an act of faith is incongruent with her characterization of herself as a hopeless cripple. When patients give away prized possessions prematurely, it may be an indirect behavioral communication that they are "putting their affairs in order" and contemplating a self-destructive act. What Mrs. Mazor least needs is validation of her decision to give Dr. Griffel the bracelet.

2. Seems consistent with several situational clues that could indicate suicidal potential. Although it is not uncommon for arthritic patients to have difficulty verbalizing their feelings, Mrs. Mazor's reference to herself as a hopeless cripple may be her way of indicating that she feels incapable of meeting the challenge of recovery and family expectations. As a result, she may be under the constant stress of a sense of failure. She expresses her tension and anxiety in a variety of ways: excessive disouragement at a time when she seems to be improving, and, incidentally, independent enough to commit the act of suicide; physical complaints of loss of appetite and sleep; a sudden episode of unusual motor behavior; changes in customary social behavior, as evidenced by her frequent visits to the solarium; and a mood change from optimism to pessimism. Also her plans to give away an item that had a great deal of meaning for her, in conjunction with the other recent behavioral changes, may be a clue that life itself has become meaningless. Her attempts to clench her fist may be a manifestation of anxiety or calm affirmation of her assessment of herself as a cripple. In this instance the technique of confrontation *might* prove invaluable in helping to protect the patient's physical safety. Although the nurse's conclusion from the implications in the situation may well be wrong, she would have no need to feel foolish or stupid. Some mistakes are fantastically creative. One fear that the nurse need not have is that broaching the subject of suicide germinates in patients ideas that never previously existed.

3. Would have some merit if two conditions prevailed. First, although there is no need to confront Mrs. Mazor with the improbability that a piece of jewelry worn around a swollen and painful wrist will suddenly cause discomfort when signs of inflammation have subsided, the nurse must not lose sight of this paradox. Second, the nurse would have to believe sincerely that the patient will improve and communicate this belief to her. Remember that the patient did not seem responsive to positive information about her condition; yet, when a patient is unable to mobilize hope by herself, she may respond to genuine interest and caring. To remind the patient of her past and present conditions and her potential for becoming may help recreate the sense of continuity needed to get a broader view of the situation. The nurse has indicated that she knows Mrs. Mazor's impaired feelings of competence have diminished her hope. This approach is a good beginning if she proceeds on the premise that life devoid of hope may also be found not worth living.

4. Would seem to be the most insightful interaction. The nurse shares her tentative assessment of the situation with the patient in a manner that communicates caring and concern. Sitting with the patient and

encouraging clarification of her self-description may facilitate understanding of the situation from Mrs. Mazor's point of view. Staying
with a troubled client also communicates a willingness to listen.
"Listening has a powerful uncovering effect" on the client, often
"pulling down protective psychological armor" as the person becomes
more open.* In this situation, patient self-disclosure seems vital to
determining whether her feelings of hopelessness, uselessness, and
unattractiveness may presage a suicidal attempt. Techniques that
foster in-depth exploration of communications of self-depreciation are
thus essential to discerning the level of nursing and medical intervention indicated, as well as to involving the patient in and validating
with her the priorities of care. Listening helps the nurse to better
coalesce the cues in the situation into a coherent picture and is a
prerequisite to correcting distortions and confirming conclusions regarding Mrs. Mazor's behavior pattern. The presence of the nurse
may communicate to individuals in submission to deep inner hurts
that they are not alone with their problems and support their attempts
to use the help that is offered.

A CRITICALLY ILL CHILD AND FAIRY TALES

Karen Foster, 5 years of age, is the apple of her parents' eyes. Karen is
a great imitator. Like her mother, she cleaned house with her own carpet
sweeper and prepared meals on a miniature stove. Karen was observant; she
noticed that her little stove did not do what the big stove in the kitchen
did—the stove that she was told never to touch. Her little stove never caused
food to sizzle or bubble, and so one morning she decided to cook breakfast
for her doll on the big stove, just as a real mommy would do. By the time
that the real mommy finished showering, the meal would be prepared. She
didn't have much to cook; her doll doesn't seem to like food anyway. Karen's
pajamas caught fire. She was admitted to the pediatric special burn unit in
critical condition. The usual measures—preventing shock and infection, applying dressings, and changing her position frequently—are written components
of the nursing care plan. Her psychosocial history states that, although she
enjoyed all activities involving locomotion, she also delighted in hearing fairy
tales. Although her physical condition is extremely precarious, Karen seems
to look forward to having her mother read stories to her. One day Mrs. Foster
tells Nurse Novak that some of the stories Karen used to delight in hearing
over and over now seem to make her visibly agitated. The mother then showed
the nurse Karen's four favorite books.

---

*From Brammer, L.: The helping relationship: process and skills, Englewood Cliffs, N.J.,
1973, Prentice-Hall, Inc., p. 27.

Which of the following four fairy tales probably provokes the *least* anxiety in Karen?

_____ 1. *Hansel and Gretel.* Two children from a poverty-stricken family are turned out of the house by their stepmother in spite of their father's protest. They become lost in the woods and finally come by chance on a witch's cottage. The witch plans a violent death for them, but the children's combined efforts lead to the witch's destruction. The children are eventually reunited with their loving father. Culpable though he was, in their absence he had vanquished the unfeeling stepmother.

_____ 2. *Little Red Riding Hood.* A delightful little girl is sent by her mother to take some food to her sick grandmother, who lives some distance away from urban developments. She is admonished not to dawdle along the way or to talk with any strangers she might meet. She disobeys and tells a wolf about her errand; he then departs to eat up the grandmother. His plans to do the same to the child when she arrives are thwarted by a woodsman. The wolf is slain and grandmother emerges intact to be reunited with Little Red Riding Hood.

_____ 3. *Three Little Pigs.* Three little pigs of indeterminate sex, have been turned out of the house by their mother and instructed to seek their fortunes. From the first day they are menaced by a wolf, who promptly succeeds in outwitting and eating two of them. In the end, the third little pig, through cleverness and fortitude, manages to lure the wolf to a death by scalding.

_____ 4. *Snow White and the Seven Dwarfs.* A beautiful, virtuous child is ordered slain by her wicked, jealous stepmother. The prospective executioner, being of faint heart, spares her life, and in the woods she eventually finds refuge in a cottage with seven little men. The stepmother manages to find and poison her into a deep sleep. She is awakened at a marriageable age by the kiss of a prince. She marries him, and they live happily ever after.

Discussion

1. Would probably be the least anxiety provoking because a child of Karen's age tends to view illness as punishment and separation as abandonment for misdeeds. This concept is reinforced in Karen's case because her hospitalization is directly related to disobeying her mother. Moreover, the 5-year-old child usually has developed a stable concept of the self as separate from the parents and must now begin to deal with the disturbing feeling that "me" could become "no me." Naturally, such agonizing thoughts are prevented as much as possible

from surfacing by denial and repression. The reality of illness is a devastating threat to the me that Karen has become. Fears of punishment, abandonment, and death, which Karen cannot voice, can be allayed in fantasy. In *Hansel and Gretel,* there are the themes of abandonment, triumph over death, and reunion with a loving parent. The children did not contribute to their own misfortune; it was beyond their control. The brother, a mothering figure, never left the little girl's side in the face of death. He protected, reassured, and took care of her. Death was outwitted, and the children returned home to a secure belonging system. All was well in the end.

2. Because of the child's wrongdoing, a mothering figure barely escaped destruction. Before being saved by the woodsman, moreover, the grandmother suffered severely. Karen is living with the consequences of her own disobedience and can probably tell that she has caused her mother grief. Seeing her mother's profound sadness may reinforce her feelings of guilt. Each time that she hears this story, she may identify with the "bad" child, and the unpleasant sensations thus aroused may be communicated in her behavior.

3. Is not comforting. For no apparent reason, death swoops down on two of the three little pigs. Only one survived. We have no way of knowing which one of the pigs Karen would identify with, but even the one that triumphed had to make strenuous efforts to do so. Karen is not strong; she hurts all over and cannot move by herself. She could not escape danger unaided. When the pigs needed them, where were the parents, the police, or other big people who are supposed to protect you? Will she eventually be left to fend for herself too? That would be impossible. Like the three little pigs, she feels imperiled from all sides—punished, possibly abandoned, and perhaps slipping into a state of nonbeing.

4. Would probably arouse a great deal of tension and anxiety in an immobilized child whose concept of time does not extend far beyond today and tomorrow. Although there are the themes of abandonment, rescue, and refuge, a deep sleep for several years must seem to her nothing less than permanent. Snow White had grown into a big girl—big enough to get married. Meanwhile, no one could help her; so she had to lie still for a long time. Karen now has something *new* to worry about: sleep can change you into a different person. Also, when you go to sleep, you do not have to awake in the morning. Sometimes seem like forever, and forever can come with sleep.

A TEENAGE EXPECTANT MOTHER—Part I

Connie Childress, a 17-year-old, single expectant mother, in her last month of pregnancy, was admitted to the antepartal unit directly from a maternity resident. The physicians at the home were concerned about Connie's sudden weight gain, elevated blood pressure, and complaints of headaches and dizziness. Her admitting diagnosis is severe preeclampsia, a condition specific to pregnancy and characterized by fluid retention, elevated blood pressure, and spillage of protein into the urine. Connie is currently the only occupant in a room usually reserved for bedfast patients. Her therapeutic regimen includes a special diet, sedation, frequent blood pressure determinations, and urinalysis four times daily. She is confined to bed except for bathroom privileges. Social service notes on the admission records indicate that Connie is estranged from her mother, who viewed her daughter's pregnancy as the latest incident in a series of "incorrigible acts," from truancy to shoplifting. Mr. Childress has had no contact with the family for several years, and the mother has always worked to support Connie and a younger sister. The Childresses are known to family court; at the mother's request and Connie's detached concurrence, it was agreed that the patient should be temporarily housed in a sheltered environment until after the birth of the baby. Social service records further indicate that Connie has made tentative plans to give her baby up for adoption. She looks more mature than her age and seems to hide behind a facade of nonchalance. She passively accepts all the nurse's ministrations and shows little interest in the therapeutic purpose of nursing and medical measures. She volunteers no personal information and tends to respond to monosyllables. When the nurses linger in the room to talk with her, Connie pops gum, thumbs through a magazine, or busies herself with filing her nails. On many occasions, however, Connie has been observed conversing animatedly with Mrs. Bradley, a middle-aged member of the housekeeping staff. Mrs. Bradley comes in every morning for such chores as dusting the furniture and cleaning the bathroom. One morning, as Miss Merril, a staff nurse, entered the room to collect a urine specimen, she apparently interrupted a serious conversation between Connie and Mrs. Bradley. Connie was speaking in lowered tones, and Mrs. Bradley was listening intently while silently patting Connie on the shoulder from time to time. When Nurse Merril greeted them, their conversation abruptly ceased. Mrs. Bradley then left the room after mentioning that she would see Connie and Nurse Merril the next day. Connie responded to the nurse's observation, "You two seem to have a lot to talk about," with, "Oh, yes, it was nothing important, you know—just about what's happening and all—you know."

Which kind of nursing intervention, would probably be the *most* appropriate in this kind of patient-care situation?

_____ 1. Nurse Merril should answer that she does not but would like to know what Connie thinks is happening and also that it might be best if Connie did not discuss personal concerns with those who do not have the professional standards, knowledge, and skills to give the help she needs.

_____ 2. Nurse Merril should arrange to speak privately with Mrs. Bradley and gently explain that Connie's personal concerns may lie beyond the scope and skills of lay persons to handle, adding that such discussions by Connie should be discouraged, since they may be inadvertently preventing the patient from using professional services.

_____ 3. Nurse Merril should mention to Connie that she would like to get to know her better and to get her opinion concerning the reasons for her early hospitalization and that to understand the situation well enough to offer more assistance, the nurse needs to find out more about how Connie feels about her current situation and the problems she perceives.

_____ 4. Nurse Merril should confer with Mrs. Bradley in privacy and suggest that she share what she has learned about the patient, so that the professional staff, who are responsible for the patient's care, can better organize their efforts to produce optimal health.

Discussion

1. May reinforce Connie's resistant attitude toward verbal problem solving. One of the developmental tasks of adolescents encompasses a need to test and rebel against authority in the process of forming an identity. Moreover, any approach based on domineering tactics would do little to help a patient whose life experience has already brought her into contact with authoritative organizations that have curtailed her autonomy with rules and regulations. One possible explanation for Connie's behavior is that, being unfamiliar with the nurse's role, she may go to great lengths to conceal her innermost thoughts from anyone perceived as part of the establishment. Patients in distress may draw comfort from many sources. Mrs. Bradley may represent an accepting mother figure to Connie, and, even though the housekeeper may not have professional credentials, she may have been exposed to life experiences similar to those of professionals and have developed "caring" qualities that help to alleviate the patient's loneliness. Also of significance is the fact that the housekeeper is one person whose daily contact with Connie is in no way threatening. Mrs. Bradley is neither going to do anything to her nor ask anything from her, and in this respect one of the barriers to communication has been automatically eliminated.

2. The nurse may be responding to her own need to dominate and control the situation rather than to the personal needs of the patient. Considerable thought needs to be given to the following questions: first, what kinds of information are essential to develop a patient-centered

plan of care; second, what are the most appropriate sources for gathering data directly related to Connie's nursing problems? Although the professional, especially if young and inexperienced, may perceive Mrs. Bradley as a threat to her goals of being "successful" in all patient interactions, there is no evidence that the nurse is impeded in acquiring information necessary for decision making. Telling Mrs. Bradley what she is equipped to handle and what she should not attempt does not resolve the nurse's communication difficulties with Connie.

Sometimes patients develop a strong sense of fellowship with identifiable members of their ethnic, religious, or economic groups. In this sense, Mrs. Bradley may have become a "significant other" in Connie's social orbit. If this is credible, the housekeeper may be helpful in facilitating Connie's adjustment to the hospital environment and eventual sharing of her concerns with other health care providers.

3. Seems to be the most appropriate because the nurse actively puts forth an effort to establish a therapeutic relationship with the patient, as well as to keep Connie's interactions with the housekeeper in the proper perspective. This approach seems to indicate that the nurse is comfortable with individual differences in patient receptivity and is secure in her professional role and competencies. Teenagers are often wary of help from authoritative figures, and their behavior may reflect a need to test the sincerity of the nurse offering help. In the third response the nurse is attempting to convey to Connie that she is interested in and available to her and that whatever is learned is for the purpose of personalizing care. Connie may need to be provided many similar opportunities before she feels comfortable enough to communicate with the nurse on levels of deep personal meaning.

4. Seems inappropriate because it is a deliberate attempt to get a nonmember of the health team to disclose information without the patient's knowledge when more relevant sources of data—the patient, social workers, others of the nursing staff, and physicians are available. Although it is essential for the nurse to coordinate all activities concerning the patient, so that helping efforts can be combined for Connie's benefit, it would seem necessary to ascertain first what each helper has to offer. Moreover, instead of seeking specific data about the patient, which incidentally could be little more than interesting gossip, Nurse Merril would do better to focus on *how* Mrs. Bradley bridged the communication gap with Connie. Perhaps the nurse can emulate some of the housekeeper's techniques and redouble her own efforts to reach the patient. More importantly Connie is beginning

to develop trust—a trust that could extend beyond the relationship with Mrs. Bradley to relationships with the staff. Rather than being interrogated, the housekeeper should be commended, so that the trust Connie is starting to manifest can be nurtured.

A TEENAGE EXPECTANT MOTHER—Part II

In spite of vigorous medical intervention, Connie's symptoms have progressed to an alarming degree, and intensive therapy with intravenous magnesium sulfate is instituted to sedate the patient and control life-threatening complications. The nurse explains to Connie that she is being transferred to a single room in which the environmental stimuli of noise, bright lights, and traffic can be better controlled. Connie is also told that the lights in her room will be dimmed and the blinds closed because rest is an important part of her treatment and these measures are being taken to help her rest. The seriousness of Connie's condition requires that trays for catheterization and special medication, a delivery pack, and suctioning and oxygen equipment be immediately available in the room. The patient's special nurse, Mrs. Phillips, helps to transfer and make her comfortable in the new setting. As Mrs. Phillips is drawing the window drapes, Connie says in a sad tone of voice, "These machines and all—I am not going to make it, am I?"

Of the following four responses, which *two* are probably the *most* supportive?

_____ 1. "You seem anxious and concerned, Connie, but I or someone else will be with you at all times. What specifically is so troubling that you think you're going to die?"

_____ 2. "This strange atmosphere and these complicated-looking machines are certainly enough to frighten anybody. Do you feel worse now than you did a few minutes ago?"

_____ 3. "From my experience, most of the equipment you see is seldom needed. Sometimes we go to such lengths to make sure that we are prepared to take every measure possible to help patients that we often frighten them."

_____ 4. "I can understand how you must be feeling. I'd be frightened too if I were in a dark room with a lot of strange equipment. I'll try to explain the purpose of the machines; then perhaps they won't be so upsetting to you."

Discussion

1. Seems to based on an inadequate appraisal of several variables in the patient-care situation. First, the patient feels acutely ill and knows that things are not going well. This knowledge is reinforced by the sudden change in her medical regimen and nursing requirements,

but, even without such external concrete evidence, remember that even some preverbal toddlers sense when they are in jeopardy. A mother who brings a toddler to the emergency ward late at night often tells the nurse that the child "acted differently," whining, clinging to her clothing and eating poorly several hours before spiking a temperature. Second, intravenous feedings are sometimes called *life water* by lay persons with the clear, although often erroneous, connotation that their condition is critical. Then, too, the patient, drowsy from sedation, has been placed in a room under conditions that simulate night. Individuals who are very ill often fear the dark of night, which symbolizes death. Consider Connie's specific focus on the oxygen and suctioning equipment. Patients know that the one thing almost all human beings do automatically and unassisted is breathing. Independent oxygenation is equated with life: the first breath is taken when one enters the world and the last when one leaves it. During the interim, oxygen therapy or its potential usage unmistakenly conveys a marked deviation from the norm and tends to support the conclusion that one is in danger. Under these circumstances, asking Connie to define reasons for her anxiety about death seems redundant.

2. Would seem to be supportive because it reflects the feeling and content of the patient's message in a manner that, if not reassuring, is least likely to add to her anxiety. Also this response shows realistic awareness that a change in Connie's condition may not be detected by direct observation. Although it is not the best therapeutic technique to answer a question with a question, sometimes factual information is best obtained from a sedated individual by limiting the answer to an unqualified yes or no.

3. Would also seem to be supportive. In this response the nurse uses a judicious amount of self-disclosure that may convey to Connie that not only is her communication understood but also her perceptions are not unusual. Although the utmost care is needed not to make the patient feel that the nurse is minimizing or dismissing the personal significance of the situation, generalizations may be a valid kind of reassurance because a threat that is known to occur in a larger segment of the patient population often loses some of its potency for the indivudual. If others have had similar experiences and recovered, so can she.

4. This attempt to familiarize the patient with the equipment in a reassuring manner may introduce more information than she can grasp. Explanations about equipment in readiness to prevent or cope with a complication that may arise must be carefully suited to the individual patient. Feedback is necessary to determine whether the information is understood. The groggy patient may be capable of

hearing only parts of the explanation; misinformation and gaps in information may be more detrimental to a sense of security than explanations that are sparse and discrete.

A TEENAGE MOTHER

Once Connie's condition was stabilized, the doctors decided that, for the safety of the mother and baby, induction of labor by Pitocin drip was necessary. Connie was delivered of a 5 pound 12 ounce baby girl, who was immediately taken to the intensive care nursery because of respiratory instability. As soon as Connie began to recover from the effects of the anesthetic, she began asking questions about the baby. She wondered whether the infant resembled her in any way, how often she would be fed, and whether she slept or cried a lot. She remarked to Nurse Phillips, "I had planned to give up the baby, but now I'm not so sure." Nurse Phillips reminded Connie that she was familiar with her plans but understood from social service that nothing was formalized as yet. Connie, continuing the conversation, added that the social workers in the hospital and the maternity home advised her that unmarried mothers who want to keep their babies are given as much assistance as possible. The patient then despairingly gave voice to the thought, "I have been wondering for quite a while whether seeing the baby would help me to make up my mind."

Which *two* of the following responses would probably be the *least* commensurate with the concepts of therapeutic communication?

_____ 1. "I can tell by your voice that you are in a low mood. If you want to see your daughter, Connie, you may, but personally I advise against it because seeing the baby is certain to cause more indecision."
_____ 2. "You seem to be experiencing a great deal of uncertainty about many things, Connie: placing your baby, keeping her, and visiting her in the nursery. What do you think we should talk about first?"
_____ 3. "I wish I had the answer, Connie, but such a far-reaching decision must be your own. We should concentrate our efforts on getting you completely well; then you may be better able to sort out the ideas and solutions that fit your life situation."
_____ 4. "I can understand why it might be difficult for you to make up your mind, Connie. Opinions vary about whether a mother should see her baby while she is contemplating adoption. I would be interested to know what you feel might happen if you saw the baby."

Discussion

1. Seems to be inappropriate advice. Counsel in the form of a considered suggestion and based on solid expertise or knowledge may have a

place in helping relationships as long as the final course of action is completely the patient's choice. Although seemingly making a direct request for information, Connie, more than likely, is asking herself a rhetorical question or thinking out loud. The decision whether to see her baby is far from inconsequential, and, according to Brammer, "advice is wholly inappropriate for dealing with major individual choice questions."* More helpful than Nurse Phillips' persuasively projecting her own ideas into the situation would be approaches that encourage exploration of Connie's indecisive feelings. Giving advice involves risks. Suggestions that do not turn out well are considered "bad advice," and the patient may blame the nurse for some of the consequent problems in her life situation.

2. May lead to a productive interaction. Nurse Phillips is attempting to help Connie gain a more definitive view of the problem and set priorities for problem solving. Encouraging the patient to choose one aspect of the problem to concentrate on may help to reduce her confusion and result in increased meaningful verbalization. Whatever tentative plans Connie made for herself and the baby prior to delivery may be vastly affected by the emotional impact of motherhood. It seems paramount that she share some of her feeling experiences before making realistically centered immediate and long-range plans. The second response also lessens the possibility that the patient will be preoccupied with one aspect of the problem and the nurse another. Should this happen, no productive exchange will be possible.

3. Does not exemplify a concept of therapeutic communication because it suggests that patients are obliging enough to separate their physical and emotional concerns into distinct segments, so that they can be dealt with one at a time. The anxiety and tension associated with the issue of seeing the baby use up energy that could be redirected to the recovery process. Therefore whatever intervention is taken to help Connie work through her feelings about the baby will inevitably promote her physical well-being.

4. Seems to be sensitive to the patient's desire to reflect on some of the probable consequences of initiating contact with the baby. Connie may think that seeing the baby will make it more difficult to give her up, or she may have a deep inner need to experience the sense of completeness and self-regard that comes from having tangible confirmation that she was able to cope with an emotionally traumatic, as well as physically life-threatening, situation from beginning to end—conception to separation. There is also some indication from

---

* From Brammer, L.: The helping relationship: process and skills, Englewood Cliffs, N.J., 1973, Prentice-Hall, Inc., p. 108.

the patient's repetitive focus on the baby that she may be planning to keep her. The nurse, by asking Connie what she *feels* might occur as a result of seeing the baby, is creating an opportunity for the patient to put strong emotions into some coherent context, since to communicate verbally, one must organize and translate mental images into understandable terminology. Nurse Phillips, acting as a sounding board for the patient to express her thoughts out loud, may better help Connie to put her feelings into perspective while she evaluates various options and outcomes. Once Connie accepts and gains some understanding of her feelings, her ability to make decisions that may lead to a healthy life for herself and the baby is likely to be enhanced.

THE PATIENT WHO ISSUES AN ULTIMATUM

Mrs. Smilen, 37 years of age, makes her initial visit to the prenatal clinic when she is 6½ months pregnant. After being examined by Dr. Gray, she is referred to the conference nurse, Miss Stein. Mrs. Smilen storms into Miss Stein's office exclaiming that she has never been treated so badly in her life! The nurse asks the patient to be seated and begins trying to find out what happened. Mrs. Smilen relates that Dr. Gray "bawled her out" for not coming to the clinic sooner, was impatient because she could not readily answer his questions concerning her three previous pregnancies, and also examined her roughly. Continuing her diatribe, Mrs. Smilen adds that the physician said her blood pressure was up and that no doubt it was, since he literally made her blood boil! Clutching her coat and purse tightly, Mrs. Smilen declares in a voice filled with fury that she will never come back to the clinic again, will stay home until her labor begins, and then will go directly to the obstetric admission unit in the hospital, since "no one around here gives a damn anyway."

Of the following four responses, which one shows the best understanding of the situation *initially?*

_____ 1. "No one intended to cause you any unpleasantness. The fact that your blood pressure is rising indicates the need for close prenatal supervision; otherwise a condition may develop to cause you difficulty later on. Feeling as strongly as you do, perhaps you can be followed up by another doctor."

_____ 2. "It is human to be upset when you think you have been unfairly treated. You say that you are angry at the doctor, but, from the tone of your voice and the way you are clutching your belongings, it seems to me that you are really taking your anger out on yourself. Think about it for a minute."

_____ 3. "It's all right to be angry; we all are sometimes. However, by refusing to return to the clinic, you will be harming yourself, not the doctor. Realistically this is such a busy clinic that Dr. Gray has probably forgotten all about the incident by this time."

_____ 4. "It would be nice if human nature were such that everyone was pleasant all the time. Your anger is understandable, but we can't always get what we want in the exact way we want it. Personalities aside, you came here today to be examined, and that's the most important thing, is it not?"

Discussion

1. Will help the patient neither to learn to handle frustrations maturely nor to adjust to some of the realities of health care settings. The important thing is to try to understand what meaning the ultimatum has for the patient. By saying that Dr. Gray bawled her out, Mrs. Smilen, in effect, may be communicating her resentment that she was treated like a child; as children so often do, she issues an ultimatum: if I can't be treated the way I want, I will punish the bad parent (physician) and make him suffer by harming myself. Furthermore, she may have expected that the nurse, in the role of the kindly parental figure, would be intimidated into yielding to the patient's unrealistic threats—which she did. Mrs. Smilen needs to be helped to see that the provocation may not have been of such great proportions as to justify her jeopardizing her personal health goals, but this approach may only communicate to the patient that her grievance is completely valid—that the doctor misbehaved and should in the future be avoided.

2. Seems to be the best initial response, since it supports the patient's emotions as valid without either sidestepping the issue or giving the appearance of taking sides in a grievance, the truth of which is unknown. By focusing on the patient's reaction, Nurse Stein candidly invites the patient to look at the harm that she is already doing herself without calling attention to her ultimatum. Mrs. Smilen may conclude that the doctor's provocation is simply not worth what she is going through and put the incident into better perspective. Once she is able to do this, she may feel freer to change her mind without experiencing a loss of face. In turn, the nurse may be able to make maximal use of her interpersonal skills in ascertaining whether some of Mrs. Smilen's anger was really a defense against the anxiety stemming from concern that the symptoms she is presenting may be serious. This kind of interviewing cannot be done until some of the negative emotions associated with the doctor-patient interaction are dissipated.

3. This attempt to get Mrs. Smilen to see how immature and even absurd her behavior may be could in fact support her belief that the doctor is unfeeling and impersonal. She will hardly be comforted by the

jarring mental image of Dr. Gray going merrily on his way, completely indifferent to her suffering. The patient's feelings of worth may be so diminished that she will indeed leave the clinic in wrath and never return.

4. Is the kind of leading question that seeks to guide Mrs. Smilen into drawing a predetermined conclusion. Instead of providing the patient an opportunity to release some of the tension associated with the interpersonal conflict, the nurse subtly communicates to the patient what her perception should be. Moreover, the patient may misinterpret this response to mean that Miss Stein is more sympathetic toward the doctor, a target of the patient's unrealistic expectations. The prenatal examination may not be the priority of care for some patients; if other needs are disregarded, the examination itself would not provide sufficient motivation to return for health supervision.

AN ABORTION EXPERIENCE

Donna and Mike, both in their early twenties, have been living together for well over a year. Donna works in a boutique and is saving money to study designing. Mike works at a garage and is currently taking courses to become a licensed mechanic. They plan to marry once Mike finishes school and is better established financially. Donna was using oral contraceptives but stopped because of the pill scare and some uncomfortable side effects. The couple decided that Mike should use condoms, but, during a time when the supply was depleted, Donna, unhappily, became pregnant. They agreed that, because of their particular circumstances, they could not sincerely commit themselves to the responsibilities of parenthood at this period in their lives, and an appointment was made for a preabortion counseling session at the local hospital center. Mike accompanied Donna to the center but said little during the interview with Nurse Whitney. However, when he wasn't mopping his brow of nonexistent perspiration, he was twisting the handkerchief in his hands. When the actual date of the scheduled abortion was being discussed, Mike blurted out, "It's all my fault; I really feel lousy about all this. What kind of a man would do this to his own kid? I just don't know, Donna. All of a sudden this doesn't feel like the right thing to do!" Donna, somewhat startled, replied in a measured tone of voice, "But, Mike, it was all settled."

Given this turn of events, which reaction by Nurse Whitney would seem to be the *most* judicious?

_____ 1. "This seems to be something that the two of you need help in working out. I will give you a referral to another member of the hospital staff who will take a look at the situation with you."

_____ 2. "This is the time when most individuals tend to have second thoughts. It is human to feel this way. It may be helpful to ventilate how you feel even if you can't resolve the problem quickly."

_____ 3. "This seems like a low point in your life, Mike, but according to recent Supreme Court rulings regarding abortion, the decision should be left to Donna and her physician."

_____ 4. "I think I understand how disturbing this must be. To whom do you turn for help when disagreements arise that seem overwhelming?"

Discussion

1. May communicate to the couple that the nurse is feeling that she is all-wise and knows what is best. Actions initiated and carried out on a patient's behalf may be perceived as manipulative when there is no element of consent. Additionally, persons should be given full explanations regarding the nature of the resource; otherwise they may reject the referral as an insult to their own problem-solving abilities or expect more than a consultant can reasonably deliver.

2. Would seem to show unwarranted confidence in the therapeutic technique of listening to people air their concerns. There are times when the nurse should not listen but prudently intervene to discourage dialogue. Such an instance would be when interpersonal conflict may exacerbate beyond the coping abilities of the participants.

3. Would be "rushing in where angels fear to tread." Emotions cannot be legislated out of existence, and citing judiciary evidence in Donna's favor may be interpreted by Mike as unwarranted interference. He may get the feeling that everyone is against him and that his opinion is worthless. The outcome might be hostility toward the nurse and hardening of his initial position. Rather than helping the couple to work out a compromise if possible, the third reaction may well cause more divisiveness.

4. Would seem to be the least inflammatory response and thus the most judicious. The nurse seems to be aware of her limitations and is attempting to involve the couple jointly in the problem-solving process. The conflict between Mike and Donna seems to have precipitated a crisis that necessitates extremely competent intervention.

COMMUNICATING WITH A PATIENT WHO CANNOT SEE

Mrs. Vaughan, married and the mother of two teenagers, is a schoolteacher in her mid-forties. She lost her eyesight after an acute, prolonged attack of glaucoma that caused irreversible damage to the optic nerve. Her medical history states that Mrs. Vaughan remembers having experienced only two earlier episodes of eye discomfort prior to her emergency admission. Because the previous symptoms of headache and colored halos around the lights lasted a relatively short time and occurred several weeks apart, the patient did not think them serious. When the doctors informed her that she had lost her vision, Mrs. Vaughan's grief was understandably profound. Much of the anger of the grieving process became intense self-loathing as the patient castigated herself for disregarding the early prodromal warnings of the condition. The patient seems overwhelmed by a sense of helplessness and hopelessness and shows no interest in being directly involved in her health care regimen. This afternoon, while Nurse Rossi is making rounds, she notices that Mrs. Vaughan is slumped down in bed with her brow furrowed and the corners of her mouth turned down. Although she seems to have managed to eat some of her dinner, the bedspread is soiled; the tray, in disarray. In response to Nurse Rossi's question, "How are things going?" the patient says nothing, but her eyes fill with tears.

Which of the following statements probably would show the best understanding by Nurse Rossi of Mrs. Vaughan's present needs?

_____ 1. "You look as if you've just about given up. This must be a really difficult time. I will set up a tray just as if I were serving you a meal. Then let's practice your feeding in privacy."

_____ 2. "You look very sad. It is natural to feel sometimes that you're not going to make it. I've known that feeling, too. Once I help you sit in the chair and feed you your dessert, you will feel a little better."

_____ 3. "I can understand that you might worry about how you'll be able to do many of the things that you used to. I have been thinking about it, too. I can obtain information about Braille to familiarize you with this method of reading if you wish."

_____ 4. "Many community resources are available to help you. You need not feel that you are all alone. Perhaps it would be a good idea for me to help you dress and walk around, so that you can get some idea of the specific services you'll need."

Discussion

1. Would probably show the best understanding of the patient's immediate needs. It is a sympathetic, positive step toward helping her achieve a sense of control over elements in her life that may seem inexorably beyond her current level of competence. Central to serious disabilities, such as blindness, is the change in body image and self-concept that plunges an individual into the depths of self-devaluation. Mrs. Vaughan needs to relearn to perform the day-to-day tasks essential to independent living—so many little things that were once routine. The longer she remains inactive and postpones facing the frustrations of adjusting to a life without sight, the greater her feelings of inadequacy and worthlessness may become. It is important for the patient to express the anger that she feels. She may be able to do this

nonverbally by banging the utensils around or perhaps by hurling the tray to the floor, or she may voice her pent-up anger directly when she is involved in the activities of daily living. However, with a great deal of support and encouragement the success that she experiences in reaching a short-range, limited goal may make her feel secure enough to begin to master skills that will help her cope with other daily challenges.

2. May offer the patient more assistance than is actually appropriate. An overprotective and overaccommodating approach may rob her of any incentive that she may have to use her own capabilities. The nurse must be aware of her own feelings, lest she sustain the patient in a state of self-pity and perpetuate a dependent relationship that Mrs. Vaughan may find difficult to relinquish.

3. Seems to show a lack of comprehension that the patient has yet to incorporate her disability into her self-concept. The nurse's efforts to help will surely fail when she prematurely suggests a substitute for sight. She needs to exercise good judgment in relation to conversation about Braille or talking books. One reason is that "if a particular item becomes a target of blanket rejection of blindness, resistance to it can crystallize and the negative attitude remain indefinite."*

4. Is also an example of planning beyond what the patient can presently appreciate. Although it is difficult for an individual to learn to cope with personal limitations without the help of outside agencies, some sightless persons prefer not to affiliate with associations for the blind. One reason that they may do so is to minimize the possibility of being stigmatized. Nurse Rossi's encouragement of the patient to ambulate would be meaningful if the purpose were to orient her to the setting and to provide an outlet for anger. Remember, however, that a depressed patient tends to walk with a slow, dragging gait because of his general state of lassitude and poor muscle tone. This typical pattern, combined with the faltering, hesitant gait of the newly blind, may exacerbate the patient's anxiety because the exercise was presented to her as a self-evaluative experience. She may get the idea that the "specific services needed" may be worse than she ever dared to fear. This image of herself would deal another blow to her self-esteem.

COMMUNICATING WITH A PATIENT WHO CANNOT HEAR

Mr. Farber, 53 years of age, is married and the father of two children. He acquired a conduction hearing loss seven years ago, in spite of surgical intervention. Prior to his disability the patient was a bus driver and is currently

---

*From Bledsoe, C. W., and Williams, R. C.: The vision needed to nurse the blind, American Journal of Nursing **66:**2432-2435, 1966.

working for the same public transportation system as a route and schedule planner. Mr. Farber was hospitalized for repair of an inguinal hernia, a condition in which a loop of the small bowel has protruded into his scrotum. The surgical ward to which the patient is admitted is an extremely busy one. Mr. Petrillo, the only professional nurse on evening duty, has delegated most of the physical aspects of the patient's preoperative care to other members of the staff. Even so, the time that he has to spend with Mr. Farber, of necessity, will be limited. Nurse Petrillo has not yet met the patient but has learned from the evening report and the Kardex that Mr. Farber communicates readily by speechreading. Mr. Petrillo had an opportunity to confer with Mr. Farber's wife and son at the conclusion of visiting hours, and they mentioned that the patient seemed apprehensive about his scheduled operation the next morning. Nurse Petrillo has been thinking of approaches that might be helpful in establishing effective communication with the patient. After discarding several ideas, he is undecided between two. When Mr. Petrillo enters the patient's room, he notes that the volume of the television set that Mr. Farber and his roommate are watching is rather high and that only the bedside lights are on in the room. After greeting both patients, the nurse explains that he would like to make a few simple environmental changes before conversing further with Mr. Farber. Once the lighting is arranged so that the patient can see him clearly, the nurse adjusts the volume of the television to lessen the possibility of his speaking in an unnatural tone of voice and misunderstanding what is said.

The two approaches that Nurse Petrillo is considering to meet the patient's needs are either to begin the discussion with social conversation or to focus more directly on his impending surgery.

Which of the following two approaches would best enhance the process of communication with the patient?

_____ 1. "Mr. Farber, several things will need to be done this evening to prepare you for surgery: skin prep, a Fleet enema, and nothing by mouth after midnight. To help you get a good night's rest, the doctor has prescribed a medication for sleep. Your family seems to think that you are anxious about the operation. Please tell me, is anything troubling you?"

_____ 2. "Mr. Farber, I understand that you work for the transportation system; my uncle does too. I would like to know what you think about all the recent layoffs? . . . Now, as to about your operation, you may already be familiar with some of the routine hospital procedures. . . ."

Discussion

1. Does not allow Mr. Farber sufficient time to familarize himself with the source of the message or to accommodate himself to the nurse's speech pattern. Speechreading involves a lot of astute guessing.

Having some idea of how words are formed on the nurse's lips and the manner in which he uses his body to convey messages helps the patient to respond more appropriately. Also helpful is giving Mr. Farber an opportunity to assimilate what has been said and to formulate a response before shifting the topic from preoperative preparations to family concerns about the patient's anxiety. Should Mr. Farber feel pressured into keeping abreast of the conversation, he may begin to doubt his ability to communicate his needs in ways that are consistent with his self-concept; and, if he feels insecure with unknown speakers, his response to the direct question, "Is anything troubling you?" will more than likely be no. In reality, his anxiety will increase if he thinks that he has received only part of a message pertinent to his welfare.

2. Would probably be the most facilitative. Social conversation is most significant to this interaction because it gives each participant an opportunity to adjust individual communication patterns under more normal circumstances. Social conversation that allows for feedback gives the patient and nurse a chance to discover and work together to overcome obstacles to clear communication. When the climate is less threatening, suggestions are less likely to be interpreted as criticism. Because the patient cannot hear the quality of his voice, he may speak in a soft monotone or too loudly. On the other hand, the nurse may need to pace his speech so that its pattern can more readily be grasped. Taking the time to make these modifications may help to ensure that the messages exchanged will be meaningful to the patient. When the nurse continues, "Now about your operation . . ." the patient is alerted to direct his attention to a different area of discussion; since he can better follow the nurse's train of thought, he may be more motivated to respond. Encouraging the patient to perceive relationships between his current and previous hospital experiences may be useful. Simply recalling past stresses with which he successfully coped may make Mr. Farber feel more in control of his present situation. If there is enough time, some discussion of the operative setting seems essential. The patient needs to be reminded that the surgical team will be masked and that he will see a great deal of movement. Deaf people tend to fear being overpowered by danger from behind. It may ease the patient's anxiety if he remembers that anesthetists customarily sit behind patient's heads and that he can anticipate being touched by persons whom he cannot see.

THE STUDENT NURSE AND MARIJUANA

Michelle and Wendy, senior nursing students in their early twenties, sponsored an engagement party for one of their classmates in Michelle's off-campus college residence. At the end of the party, the group decided to continue feting the guest of honor at the local pub. Michelle and Wendy opted to stay behind and tidy up a bit before joining them. After the others had left, Michelle suggested that she and Wendy take time out to unwind and "turn on" before attacking the disorder. Michelle then went on to say that she would let Wendy in on a little secret if she would promise to keep it "under her hat." Michelle then left the room and returned with several short, thin cigarettes, which she identified as "pot." In response to Wendy's protests, Michelle explained that "Mary Janes" were a harmless but enjoyable way to relax and added that when she smoked them, the "high" was a perfect antidote to the stress of endless studying and the weariness of keeping up with assignments. Michelle added that, as a matter of fact, marijuana was less harmful than the highballs Wendy drank and the cigarettes she usually smoked. Michelle then reclined on the sofa and with eyes closed lit up and began inhaling deeply on a stick of pot, meanwhile telling Wendy not to knock it until she tried it.

Wendy does not approve of the practice; under these circumstances, which of her decisions would probably involve the *least* "appropriate actions?"

_____ 1. Wendy, firmly but kindly, should tell Michelle that, even though she would like to stay, unless Michelle disposes of the marijuana at once, she will leave, rather than continue witnessing what is clearly an unlawful practice.

_____ 2. Wendy should let Michelle know that she is sorry but that she cannot keep secret a practice that is potentially detrimental to her friend's health and professional career and that, to help her, this infraction of the professional code must be reported.

_____ 3. Wendy should point out to Michelle that the use of drugs to soften difficulties is often a plea for help and suggest that her friend seek guidance as soon as possible from a member of the nursing faculty to whom she feels that she can speak freely.

_____ 4. Wendy should candidly exchange ideas with Michelle about the use of drugs in general, point out that they both need further enlightenment, and explore the possibility of getting the student nursing club to sponsor seminars led by experts in the field.

Discussion

1. May be appropriate, depending on the value Michelle places on the friendship and whether she perceives Wendy's ultimatum to be motivated by genuine concern, rather than self-interest. Otherwise, even if this assertive approach accomplishes the short-range goal of getting Michelle to refrain from smoking marijuana in Wendy's presence,

it may sabotage efforts to engage Michelle in dialogue concerning her choice and its consequences. Although the risk of being discovered under the presented circumstances may not be great, the serious legal and social sanctions against the possession and use of marijuana cannot be lightly dismissed. Realistically, should Michelle's behavior come to the direct attention of authorities, the possibility exists that in a legal proceeding Wendy would be compelled to disclose information about the episode or face contempt of court. However, having a friend set limits and then show a willingness to listen may offer Michelle a significant opportunity to explore her feelings and behavior more fully and provide some motivation for learning to modify her behavior, tastes, and ideas.

2. Seems to be the *least* appropriate action, but Wendy's intent is not faulted, for it is true that marijuana is a mild hallucinogen whose long-term physiologic and psychologic effects have yet to be determined. Although laws concerning the possession and use of marijuana vary from state to state, not easily disregarded is the conclusion by Lipp and co-workers that "medical personnel who use marijuana face frightening legal hazards and career risks of considerable proportions such as jeopardizing a student's chance for graduation, state licensure and employment."* The reason that this approach is wrong has profound implications for both personal and professional relationships; that is, neither a colleague nor a patient should be misled to believe that confidential information is safe when in fact it is not. Honesty in human relationships requires that the listener not remain riveted in the face of revelations but urge restraint whenever possible before privileged information is divulged. Wendy had ample time to warn Michelle of her ethical stance prior to the actual incident. The argument that confidences should not be honored when an illegal act is being committed or contemplated may be valid, but one needs also to keep in mind that the communicant of a secret should be given the outright choice to keep incriminating information to himself or to disclose it and take his chances. It is hypocritical to react later as if one were unfairly manipulated into becoming part of a secret pact. Central to the concept of confidentiality is sensitivity to the fact that much harm may be done in the name of help, as well as awareness that only information relevant to the fundamental safety and welfare of the secret sharer and others should be communicated through the channels of authority. Moreover, in this regard, if Wendy were truly convinced that her friend's critical faculties were being impaired,

---

*From Lipp, M., Benson, S., and Allen, P.: Marijuana use by nurses and nursing students, American Journal of Nursing **71**:2339-2341, 1971.

in Michelle's and her patients' best interest, naturally Wendy would have no recourse but to communicate her concern to those in a position to help.

3. Begins with a point of view that already Michelle, in a way, has refuted. Even so, the use of such drugs as alcohol and cigarettes by Wendy does not carry the same social proscriptions as the use of marijuana. By recognizing that her friend may need more help than she can give, Wendy suggests a course of action and places the responsibility for following through where it properly belongs, with Michelle. More importantly, there may be a feeling tone in this approach that communicates to Michelle that Wendy sincerely wants to use what she has learned about Michelle for and not against her.

4. May give impetus to a mutually problem-solving enterprise, launched by acknowledgments of human frailty and aboveboard dialogue that is tolerant of contrary opinions. Marijuana, like other cigarettes, may be available for a long time, and in neither instance does inner motivation to abstain from its use seem strengthened by the fear of legal or medical outcomes. Student nurses are a heterogeneous group and part of the dominant culture that believes commercial promises of "better living through chemistry" and that intrinsic to the good life is instant relief of tension and anxiety. During the interim between childhood and adulthood, youth tends to seek greater independence from parental and other authority figures, but there remains the intense human need to belong, which, in turn, may foster more reliance on peer relationships for status, as well as understanding. Thus peer relationships, in contrast to strictly professional interactions, may provide the setting for receptivity to influential points of view, as well as for learning experiences to which students may better relate. Furthermore, although the opposite is certainly true, peer relationships may be powerful stimuli for making *self-enhancing* choices that may help bridge the gap between dreams and reality with mature behavior.

Bibliography

American Hospital Association: A patient's bill of rights, Chicago, 1972, The Association.

Beauchamp, J.: Euthanasia and the nurse practitioner, 1975, Nursing Forum 14:56-73, 1975.

American Nurses' Association Committee on Ethical, Legal and Professional Standards: Code for nurses with interpretive statements, Kansas City, Mo., 1976, The Association.

Committee on Psychiatry and Law. In The right to abortion: a psychiatric view, New York, 1970, Charles Scribner's Sons.

1973 convention issues: proposed resolution No. 1 on rights and responsibilities in nursing practice, Michigan Nurse Newsletter 46:26, Sept., 1973.

Cornish, J.: Women's experiences with abortion. In McNall, L. K., and Galeener, J. T.: Current practice in obstetric and gynecologic nursing, St. Louis, 1976, The C. V. Mosby Co.

Dedek, J.: Human life: some moral issues, New York, 1972, Sheed & Ward, Inc.

Fagin, C.: Nurses' rights, American Journal of Nursing 75:82-85, 1975.

Fletcher, J.: Ethics and euthanasia, American Journal of Nursing 73:670-675, 1973.

Foote, E.: The role of law (and lawyers) in medicine, Washington University Magazine 46:26-30, Spring, 1976.

Goldstein, T.: Death and the law, The New York Times, p. 38, April 2, 1976.

Halley, M., and Harvey, W.: Medical vs. legal definitions of death, Journal of the American Medical Association 204:423-425, 1968.

Hershey, N.: students as staff nurses? American Journal of Nursing 67:117, 1967.

Hilger, T.: The medical hazards of legally induced abortion. In Hilger, T., and Horan, D., editors: Abortion and social justice, New York, 1972, Sheed & Ward, Inc.

Horty, J.: Law and the courts, Modern Hospital 120:33-34, June, 1973.

Lader, L.: Abortion II: making the revolution, Boston, 1973, Beacon Press.

Lanahan, C.: Anxieties and fears of patients seeking abortion. In McNall, L. K., and Galeener, J. T.: Current practice in obstetric and gynecologic nursing, St. Louis, 1976, The C. V. Mosby Co.

LeRoux, R., Barnes, S., Gottesfeld, K., West, D., and Tolch, M.: Abortion, American Journal of Nursing 70:1919-1925, 1970.

Mecklenburg, F.: The indications for induced abortion. In Hilger, T., and Horan, D., editors: Abortion and social justice, New York, 1972, Sheed & Ward, Inc.

Meyers, D.: The legal aspects of euthanasia, Bioscience 23:467, Aug., 1973.

Morrison, R.: Dying, Scientific American 229:55-60, 1973.

Osofsky, H., and Osofsky, J., editors: The abortion experience: psychological and medical impact, New York, 1973, Harper & Row, Publishers.

Paulen, A.: Living with cancer: the rights of the patient and the rights of the nurse. In Peterson, B., and Kellogg, C., editors: Current practice in oncologic nursing, vol. 1, St. Louis, 1976, The C. V. Mosby Co.

Quinn, N., and Somers, A.: The Patient's Bill of Rights: a significant aspect of the consumer revolution, Nursing Outlook 22:240-244, 1974.

Quint, J.: Obstacles to helping the dying,

American Journal of Nursing **66**:1568-1571, 1966.

Ramsey, P.: Reference points in deciding about abortion. In Noonan, J., editor: The morality of abortions, Cambridge, Mass., 1972, Harvard University Press.

Sanders, M., and Fisher, J.: The crisis in American medicine, New York, 1961, Harper & Row, Publishers.

Shainess, N.: Abortion and psychiatry. In Hall, R., editor: Abortion in a changing world, vol. 2, New York, 1968, Columbia University Press.

Shindell, S.: The law in medical practice, Pittsburgh, 1966, University of Pittsburgh Press.

Silva, M.: Science, ethics, and nursing, American Journal of Nursing **74**:2004-2007, 1974.

Smith, D.: Some ethical considerations in caring for the dying. In American Nurses' Association clinical sessions, New York, 1975, Appleton-Century-Crofts.

Smith, H.: Ethics and new medicine, Nashville, Tenn., 1970, Abingdon Press.

Still, J.: The levels of life and semantic confusion, ETC **28**:9-21, March, 1971.

Stockhouse, M.: Abortion and animation. In Hall, R., editor: Abortion in a changing world, vol. 2., New York, 1968, Columbia University Press, p. 57.

Sudnow, D.: Passing on, Englewood Cliffs, N.J., 1976, Prentice-Hall, Inc., p. 84.

The dying person's bill of rights, American Journal of Nursing **75**:98-101, 1975.

Vaughn, P.: The pill turns twenty, The New York Times Magazine, p. 9+, June 13, 1976.

Weber, L.: Ethics and euthanasia: another view, American Journal of Nursing **73**:1228-1231, 1973.

White, R.: Abortion and psychiatry. In Hall, R., editor: Abortion in a changing world, vol. 2, New York, 1968, Columbia University Press.

Index

A

Abortion, 167-180
  case study of, 241-242
  and "conscience clause," 167
  and considerations for human life, 169
  and euthanasia, 151-182
    code for nurse concerning, 151-154
  and father of unborn child, 177
  and forcible conception, 174
  and incest, 174
  and intrauterine transfusion, 169
  and mental health of mother, 176
  and morality, 168-171
  positions for and against, 170
  and rape, 174
  stigmatization of, 169
  and suicidal ideation, 176
  and unwanted pregnancy, 174-177
  and "women's rights," 169
Acceptance in grief process of dying person, 120
Adler, A., 22
Adolescence and identity vs. identity diffusion, 102-103; *see also* Childhood
Adulthood
  and generativity vs. self-absorption, 104-105
  young, intimacy vs. isolation in, 103-104
Advocate, patient's, 7
Aguilera, D., 112
Aiken, J., 195
Aiken, L., 195
Alcoholism, case study of, 222-224
Allen, P., 248
American Hospital Association, 155
Amputation and body image, 130
Anger in grief process of dying person, 120
Anomic suicide, 97
Antiabortion positions, 170
Antidepressants, 100
  nonprescription, and young adult, 104

Antisocial behavior and sickness, 43
Anxiety, 84-89
  depression, and stages of man, 100-106
  differences between, and depression, 99-100
  mechanism of, 37
  nursing intervention in, 88-89
  and pain, 51
  and sickness, 43
Apathy, 21
Appearance
  and depression, 93-94
  and obesity, 145
Art and communication, 8-12
Assessment, 9-10
Autonomy vs. shame in early childhood, 101
Awareness, types of, of dying person, 120

B

Bargaining in grief process of dying person, 120, 121-122
Behavior
  antisocial, and sickness, 43
  characteristic, of those needing help, 83-107
  defensive, 85-88
Behavior modification and language behavior, 38
Behavioral theories, relationship of, to communication, 34-35
Behaviorism; *see* Behavioristic theory
Behavioristic theory, 35, 37-38
Belonging, need for, of Maslow, 56
Benson, S., 248
Bereaved, helping, 114-117
Bill of rights; *see* Rights
Biologic death, definition of, 159
Birth, communication at, 8
Birth control, 174-177

252

Harvard Medical School, definition of death of, 160
Healer, energy flow from, to patient, 49
Healing
  and parapsychology, 49
  and touch, 68
Hearing
  and dying person, 160
  loss of, 139-142; *see also* Deafness
    communication with patient with, case study of, 244-246
    and depression, 141
    and fear of being misunderstood, 140-141
    and finger spelling, 140
    and lipreading, 140
    and loneliness, 135
    partial, 142-143
    and sign language, 140
    and speechreading, 140
Heart disease, 132
Hector, W., 225
Help, characteristic behaviors of those needing, 83-107
Helper, nurse as, 29-30
Helping, 12-13
Helping skills, application of, to selected crises, 109-125
Honesty, 19-20
Hospitalization
  and identity, 42-43
  and obesity, 147
Hostility and suicide, 96
Human beings, theoretical assumptions concerning nature of, 33-53
Human nature, five perspectives of, 35-52
Human needs, five basic, of Maslow, 45-46
Human rights; *see* Rights
Humaneness, definition of, 154
Humanism; *see* Humanistic theory
Humanistic theory, 35, 44-47
Humanness, definition of, 154
Humor, 25-28
Hypertension, case study of, 208-211
Hypocrisy, 17

I

Id, 36-37, 41, 43, 44
Ideal self in role theory, 40, 41-42
Identification, 86
Identity
  diffusion of, vs. identity in adolescence, 102-103
  and hospitalization, 42-43

Identity—cont'd
  vs. identity diffusion in adolescence, 102-103
Ileostomy, case study of, 216-219
Illness, social role of, 42-44
Implementation phase of assessment, 10
Incest and abortion, 174
Individuality as right of dying person, 157
Industry vs. inferiority in school age of childhood, 102
Infancy, trust vs. mistrust in, 100-101
Inferiority vs. industry in school age of childhood, 102
Inheritance, role of, and obesity, 145
Initiative vs. guilt in play age of childhood, 101-102
Instinct, death and life, 36
Instinctual drive, 37
Integrity vs. despair and old age, 105-106
International Planned Parenthood Federation, 178
Interpersonal communication, 56
Interpersonal relationship, 16
  definition of, 28-29
  and depression, 94
  exercises in, 183-249
  and nursing, 4
  right of nurse to create, with patient, 156
Intervention
  crisis; *see* Crisis intervention
  nursing; *see* Nursing
Interview
  body language in, 63-66
  eye contact in, 63-65
  face-to-face arrangement in, 63-64
  setting of, 61-62
  therapeutic communication as, 57
Intimacy vs. isolation in young adulthood, 103-104
Intrauterine device, 173
Intrauterine transfusion and abortion, 169
Introjection, 86
Intuition, 9, 48
Involuntary euthanasia; *see* Euthanasia, involuntary
Involutional melancholia, 105
Involvement and loneliness, 135
Irwin, T., 101
Isolation
  vs. intimacy in young adulthood, 103-104
  and pain, 52
IUD; *see* Intrauterine device

J

Jourard, S. M., 59, 220

Nurse—cont'd
noninvolvement of, 155
obligation of, 152
rights of, 154-159
student, and marijuana, case study of, 246-249
uniform of, 61
visiting, and fee setting, case study of, 188-191
Nurse-doctor conflict, case study of, 208-211
Nurse-patient relationship, communication as core of, 12-16
Nursing; *see also* Nurse
and anxiety, 88-89
contact with people in, 13-14
and depersonalization, 6-7
and family, 3, 8
and feelings, 14
future of, 30
and generalization to "massness," 7-8
and grief of bereaved person, 116-117
and interpersonal relations, 4
and knowledge, 15
and loss of sight, 138-139
process of, right of patient to, 155
and "psychological mothering," 16
and shared relationship with patient, 14
as social service, 13
and specialization, 6-7
and suicide, 98-99
and totality of involvement, 14
and touching, 6
Nursing assistants, 4
Nursing intervention; *see* Nursing
Nurturing, 12
Nutrition, teaching, case study of, 186-188

O

Obesity, 143-148
and appearance, 145
and body image, 147
and compulsive eating, 146
and depression, 146-147
and gluttony, 144
as habituation syndrome, 147-148
and hospitalization, 147
and jolly fat man stereotype, 147
and number of fat cells in infancy, 145
and role of inheritance, 145
satisfaction of emotions with food in, 146
and self-contempt, 144
Oedipal desires, 101
Open question, 75-78
Open-ended statement, 76

Organic pain of dying person, 122
Orlando, I., 13, 78
Overcompensation, 87

P

Pain, 50-52
and anxiety, 51
and attention, 51
of dying person, 122-123
and emotional state of patient, 51
and euthanasia, 164
and isolation, 52
and night, 51-52
organic, of dying person, 122
psychic, of depression of dying person, 122
and sociocultural factors, 51
Parad, H., 110
Paranormal phenomena, 47-50
Paraphrasing, use of, 78-79
Parapsychology, 47-50
Patient
advocate of, 7
communication and personality of, 11
crying, case study of, 216-219
demanding, case study of, 193-197
energy flow from healer to, 49
informing, about diagnosis, 19-20
informing, about prognosis, 19-20
needs of, and therapeutic communication, 56-57
personality of, and nursing, 11
rights of, 154-159
self-expression of, 11
with venereal disease, case study of, 199-203
who fears life more than death, case study of, 219-222
who issues ultimatum, case study of, 239-241
who makes sexual overtures, case study of, 203-208
Patient confessions, 71
Patient-nurse relationship, 16, 60-61
termination of, 28-29
Paulen, A., 156
People, contact with, in nursing, 13
Peplau, H., 12-13, 15-16
Personality, changes in, and sickness, 43
Phantom limb phenomenon, 130
Physiologic needs of Maslow, 45, 61
Pill, contraceptive, 173
Pity, 23
Placebo effect, 52
Planning phase of assessment, 10
Pleasure principle, 36